CW00832391

Oral Medicine
Update for the Dental Team

Production Editor: Stephen Hancocks
Designer: Lisa Dunbar

Oral Medicine
Update for the Dental Team

Dr Jane Luker

Jane Luker is Postgraduate Dental Dean for South West England having previously been a Consultant in Dental and Maxillofacial Radiology. From 2002-2009 she was Clinical Director/Lead Doctor for Dental Services in Bristol and is currently President of the British Society of Dental & Maxillofacial Radiology. Additionally Jane is an examiner in the Diploma of Dental Radiology, Royal College of Radiologists.

Professor Crispian Scully CBE

Crispian Scully is Director of the WHO Collaborating Centre for Oral Health-General Health, President of the British Society for Oral Medicine and holds a string of positions, awards and honours in relation to his career in oral medicine and associated specialties. Crispian has been Dean at the University of Bristol and UCL and is immediate past-President of the International Academy of Oral Oncology.

Dr David Felix

David Felix is the Postgraduate Dental Dean for Scotland and was an elected Council member of the British Society for Oral Medicine from 1991, serving as Honorary Secretary/Treasurer from 1994 – 2002 and President from 2003 – 2005. David maintains an active contribution to the peer reviewed literature with publications on oral medicine and more recently on postgraduate training and education.

Series Editor
F.J. Trevor Burke
Professor of Dental Primary Care
University of Birmingham School of Dentistry

DentalUpdate Books

©2015, Stephen Hancocks Limited. All rights reserved.

The right of Jane Luker, Crispian Scull and David Felix to be identified as authors of this work has been asserted by them in accordance with teh Copyright, Designs and Patents Act 1988.

No part of this publication may be reproduced, stored in a retrieval system, or transmitted in any form or by any means, electronic, mechanical, photocopying, recording or otherwise, without either the prior permission of the publishers or a licence permitting restricted copying in the United Kingdom issued by the Copyright Licensing Agency, 90 Tottenham Court Road, London W1T 4LP. Permissions may be sought directly from Stephen Hancocks Limited, Little Steine, Hill Farm Lane, Duns Tew, Oxon OX25 6JH. Telephone Number: 01869 347839. (http://www.shancocksltd.co.uk)

First published 2015

ISBN 978-0-9932280-0-1

British Library Cataloguing in Publication Data
A catalogue record for this book is available from the British Library

Note
Medical knowledge is constantly changing. As new information becomes available, changes in treatment, procedures, equipment and the use of drugs become necessary. The authors and the publishers have taken care to ensure that the information given in the text is accurate and up to date. However, readers are strongly advised to confirm that the information, especially with regard to drug usage, complies with the latest legislation and standards of practice.

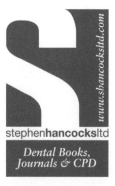

stephenhancocksltd
*Dental Books,
Journals & CPD*

DentalUpdate Books

Printed in the United Kingdom

Contents

Acknowledgements

Our thanks to all the patients, nurses, students and colleagues who have assisted and supported us, and our families for tolerating the loss of time resulting from this work.

Preface

Through this book we hope to educate and inspire each member of the dental team in the main points and relevance in healthcare of Oral Medicine in a practical way, indicating disease aetiopathogenesis, clinical features, diagnosis and patient management. The book is based on a recent series of articles in *Dental Update* and should prove of value to the whole dental healthcare team. The information in the bookwill also be helpful to the whole healthcare team as dental education is typically lacking for doctors, nurses and pharmacists who may be called upon to advise on oral issues.

Improved social and medical care has increased the life span of many people, including those with previously life-threatening disorders. New and emerging infections (e.g. HIV) and iatrogenic issues (e.g. new drugs, immunosuppressive treatment, cancer therapy) are increasingly seen. Many of these people are vulnerable to the common and novel oral diseases and require special attention. It is thus important that adequate attention is paid both to medical, drug and social history. It is important to apply preventive programmes and educate patients and parents in hygiene to minimise the risk of oral infections.

We warmly acknowledge the guidance and help of Stuart Thompson, Stephen Hancocks, Trevor Burke and Angela Stroud in helping us to bring this project to fruition.

The quality of care that patients receive is paramount, this includes, patient experience, patient outcomes and patient safety. Use of medical history questionnaires is good practice only if the information is utilised correctly as in any check list. It is important to ensure that you are familiar with a patient's full medical and drug history prior to prescribing any medication and to have valid patient consent. Contraindications must always be checked and the patient warned of any possible adverse effects.

The information in this book has been carefully checked but neither the authors nor publisher can accept any legal responsibility for any errors or omissions that may be made. Neither the authors nor publisher makes any warranty, expressed or implied, with respect to material herein.

DHF, C.S. J.L
Edinburgh, London & Bristol
2015

Ulcers: Aphthous and other Common Ulcers

1

1. Ulceration

Ulceration is a breach in the oral epithelium, which typically exposes nerve endings in the underlying lamina propria, resulting in pain or soreness, especially on eating spicy foods or citrus fruits. Patients vary enormously in the degree to which they suffer and complain of soreness in relation to oral ulceration. It is always important to exclude serious disorders such as oral cancer (Article 3) or other serious disease, but not all patients who complain of soreness have discernible organic disease. Even in those with detectable lesions, the level of complaint can vary enormously – some patients with large ulcers complain little; others with minimal ulceration complain bitterly of discomfort. Sometimes there is a psychogenic or cultural influence.

Terminology

Epithelial thinning or breaches may be seen in:

■ Mucosal atrophy or desquamation – terms often used for thinning of the epithelium which assumes a red appearance since the underlying lamina propria containing blood vessels shows through. Most commonly seen in desquamative gingivitis (usually related to lichen planus, or less commonly to pemphigoid) and in geographic tongue (erythema migrans, benign migratory glossitis), a similar process may also be seen in systemic disorders such as deficiency states (of iron, folic acid or B vitamins).
■ Mucosal inflammation (mucositis, stomatitis) can cause soreness. Viral stomatitis, candidosis, radiation mucositis, chemotherapy-related mucositis and graft-versus-host-disease are examples.
■ Erosion is the term used for superficial breaches of the epithelium. These often initially have a red appearance, since there is little damage to the underlying lamina propria, but it typically becomes covered by a fibrinous exudate and then has a yellowish appearance (Figure 1). Erosions are common in vesiculobullous disorders such as pemphigoid.
■ Ulcer is the term used usually where there is damage both to epithelium and lamina propria. An inflammatory halo, if present, also highlights the ulcer with a red halo, around the yellow or grey ulcer (Figure 2). Most ulcers are due to local causes such as trauma or burns but recurrent aphthous stomatitis must always be considered.

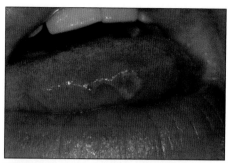

Figure 1. A small erosion.

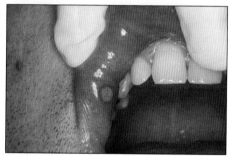

Figure 2. Minor aphthous ulcer, labial mucosa.

Causes of oral ulceration

Ulcers and erosions can also be the final common manifestation of a spectrum of conditions, ranging from epithelial damage resulting from trauma, to an immunological attack as in lichen planus, pemphigoid or pemphigus, to damage because of an immune defect, as in HIV disease and leukaemia, infections as in herpesviruses, tuberculosis and syphilis, or nutritional defects such as in vitamin deficiencies and some gastrointestinal disease (Tables 1 and 2).

Ulcers of local causes

At any age, there may be burns from chemicals of various kinds, heat, cold, or ionizing radiation or factitious ulceration, especially of the maxillary gingivae (Figures 3 and 4).

Children may develop ulceration of the lower lip by

accidental biting following dental local anaesthesia. Ulceration of the upper labial fraenum, especially in a child

Causes	Mnemonic
Systemic diseases	**So**
Malignant disease	**Many**
Local causes	**Laws**
Aphthae	**And**
Drugs	**Directives**

Table 1. Main causes of oral ulceration.

with bruised and swollen lips, or subluxed teeth or fractured jaw can represent non-accidental injury. At any age, trauma, hard foods, or appliances may also cause ulceration. The lingual fraenum may be traumatized by repeated rubbing over the lower incisor teeth in cunnilingus or in recurrent coughing as in whooping cough or in self-mutilating conditions.

Most ulcers of local cause have an obvious aetiology, are acute, usually single ulcers, last less than 3 weeks and heal spontaneously. Chronic trauma may produce an ulcer with a keratotic margin (Figure 5).

Systemic disease
Blood (Haematological) disorders
    Anaemia
    Gammopathies
    Haematinic deficiencies
    Leukaemia and myelodysplastic syndrome
    Neutropenia and other white cell dyscrasias
Infections
    Acute necrotizing gingivitis
    Chickenpox
    Deep mycoses
    Hand, foot and mouth disease
    Herpangina
    Herpes simplex virus
    HIV
    Infectious mononucleosis
    Syphilis
    Tuberculosis
Gastrointestinal disease
    Coeliac disease
    Crohn disease
    Ulcerative colitis
Skin (Mucocutaneous) disease
    Behcet syndrome
    Chronic ulcerative stomatitis
    Epidermolysis bullosa
    Erythema multiforme
    Lichen planus
    Pemphigus vulgaris
    Sub-epithelial immune blistering diseases
    (pemphigoid and variants, dermatitis
    herpetiformis linear IgA disease),

Malignant neoplasms
    Oral
    Encroaching from antrum

Local causes
    Trauma
        Appliances
        Iatrogenic
        Non-accidental injury
        Self-inflicted
        Sharp teeth or restorations
    Burns
        Chemical
        Cold
        Electric
        Heat
        Radiation
Aphthae
Drugs
    Cytotoxic drugs
    Nicorandil
    NSAIDs

Miscellaneous uncommon diseases
    Eosinophilic ulcer
    Giant cell arteritis
    Hypereosinophilic syndrome
    Lupus erythematosus
    Necrotizing sialometaplasia
    Periarteritis nodosa
    Reiter syndrome
    Sweet syndrome
    Wegener granulomatosis

Table 2. Main causes of mouth ulcers.

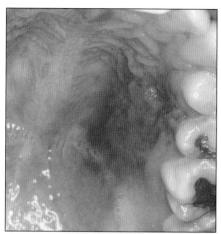

Figure 3. Thermal burn, palate.

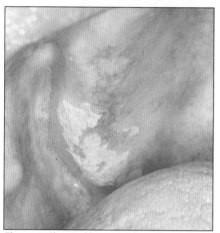

Figure 4. Chemical burn, right maxillary tuberosity.

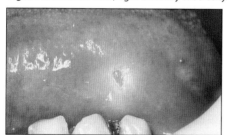

Figure 5. Traumatic ulceration, lateral tongue.

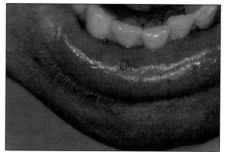

Figure 6. Minor aphthous ulceration.

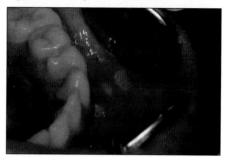

Figure 7. Minor aphthous ulceration.

Recurrent aphthous stomatitis (RAS; aphthae; canker sores) RAS is a very common condition which typically starts in childhood or adolescence and presents with multiple recurrent small, round or ovoid ulcers with circumscribed margins, erythematous haloes, and yellow or grey base (Figures 6 and 7).

RAS affects at least 20% of the population, with the highest prevalence in higher socio-economic classes. Virtually all dentists will see patients with aphthae.

Aetiopathogenesis

Immune mechanisms appear at play in a person with a genetic predisposition to oral ulceration. A genetic predisposition is present, and there is a positive family history in about one third of patients with RAS. Immunological factors are also involved, with T helper cells predominating in the RAS lesions early on, along with some natural killer (NK) cells. Cytotoxic cells then appear in the lesions and there is evidence for an antibody dependent cellular cytotoxicity (ADCC) reaction. It now seems likely therefore that a minor degree of immunological dysregulation underlies aphthae.

RAS may be a group of disorders of different pathogeneses. Cross-reacting antigens between the oral mucosa and micro-organisms may be the initiators, but attempts to implicate a variety of bacteria or viruses have failed.

Predisposing factors

Most people who suffer RAS are otherwise apparently completely well. In a few, predisposing factors may be identifiable, or suspected. These include:
■ Stress: underlies RAS in many cases. RAS is typically worse at examination times;
■ Trauma: biting the mucosa, and dental appliances may

lead to some ulcers;
- Haematinic deficiency (deficiencies of iron, folic acid (folate) or vitamin B_{12}) in up to 20% of patients;
- Sodium lauryl sulphate (SLS), a detergent in some oral healthcare products, may produce oral ulceration;
- Cessation of smoking: may precipitate or aggravate RAS;
- Gastrointestinal disorders particularly coeliac disease (gluten-sensitive enteropathy) and Crohn's disease in about 3% of patients;
- Endocrine factors in some women whose RAS is clearly related to the fall in progestogen level in the luteal phase of their menstrual cycle;
- Immune deficiency; ulcers of a similar appearance to RAS may be seen in HIV and other immune defects, although clearly the aetiopathogenesis is different;
- Food allergies: in some studies hypersensitivity to various food additives has been shown to be important, although this is not a universal finding.

Drugs (see below), Behcet syndrome, HIV, Epstein-Barr virus, auto-inflammatory states (periodic fevers) and skin diseases, such as erythema multiforme, may occasionally produce aphthous-like lesions.

Keypoints: aphthous ulcers

- They are so common that all the dental team will see them;
- It is important to rule out predisposing causes (sodium lauryl sulphate, certain foods/drinks, stopping smoking or vitamin or other deficiencies) or conditions such as Behcet syndrome that can cause aphthous-like lesions;
- It is necessary therefore to enquire about eye, genital, gastrointestinal or skin lesions and fever;
- Topical corticosteroids are the main treatment.

Clinical features

There are three main clinical types of RAS, though the significance of these distinctions is unclear and it is conceivable that they may represent three different diseases.

1. Minor aphthous ulcers (MiAU; Mikulicz Ulcer)

- Occur mainly in the 10–40 year age group;
- Often cause minimal symptoms;
- Are small round or ovoid ulcers 2–4mm in diameter in most situations but often more linear when in the buccal sulcus, a common site. The ulcer base is initially yellowish but assumes a greyish hue as healing and epithelialization proceeds. They are surrounded by an erythematous halo and some oedema;
- Are found mainly on the non-keratinized mobile mucosa of the lips, cheeks, floor of the mouth, sulci or ventrum of the tongue.

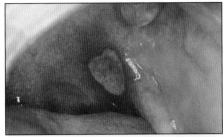

Figure 8. Major aphthous ulceration, soft palate complex.

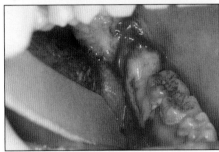

Figure 9. Major aphthous ulceration.

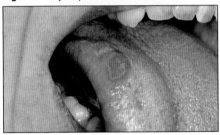

Figure 10. Major aphthous ulceration.

They are only uncommonly seen on the keratinized mucosa of the palate or dorsum of the tongue;
- Occur in groups of only a few ulcers (1–6) at a time;
- Heal in 7–10 days;
- Recur at intervals of 1–4 months;
- Leave little or no evidence of scarring

2. Major aphthous ulcers (MjAU; Sutton's Ulcers; Periadenitis Mucosa Necrotica Recurrens (PMNR)) (Figures 8, 9, 10)

- Are larger, of longer duration, of more frequent recurrence, and often more painful than minor ulcers;
- MjAUs are round or ovoid like minor ulcers, but they are larger and associated with surrounding oedema;
- Reach a large size, usually about 1 cm in diameter or even larger;
- Are found on any area of the oral mucosa, including the keratinized dorsum of the tongue or palate;
- Occur in groups of only a few ulcers (1–6) at one time;

- Heal slowly over 10–40 days;
- Recur extremely frequently;
- May heal with scarring;
- Occasionally found with a raised erythrocyte sedimentation rate or plasma viscosity.

3. Herpetiform ulceration (HU)

- Are found in a slightly older age group than the other forms of RAS;
- Are found mainly in females;
- Begins with vesiculation which passes rapidly into multiple minute pinhead-sized discrete ulcers (Figure 11);
- Involve any oral site including the keratinized mucosa, increase in size and coalesce to leave large round ragged ulcers;
- Heal in 10 days or longer;
- Are often extremely painful;
- Recur so frequently that ulceration may be virtually continuous;
- Despite the name they have nothing to do with herpes infection.

Diagnosis

There are no specific tests, so the diagnosis must be made on history and clinical features alone. However, to exclude the systemic disorders discussed above, it is often useful to undertake the investigations shown in Table 3.

Biopsy is rarely indicated, usually where a different diagnosis is suspected.

Management

Other similar disorders, such as Behcet syndrome, must be ruled out (Article 2). Predisposing factors should then be corrected. Fortunately, the natural history of RAS is one of eventual remission in most cases. However, few patients have spontaneous remission until after several years and, although there is no curative treatment, measures should be taken to relieve symptoms and reduce ulcer duration.
- Good oral hygiene should be maintained. Chlorhexidine or triclosan mouthwashes may help.

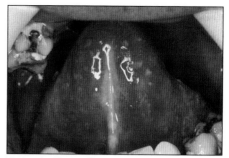

Figure 11. Herpetiform aphthae.

- Full blood count;
- Haematinics;
  - Ferritin;
  - Folate;
  - Vitamin B_{12};
- Serological screen for coeliac disease (tissue transglutaminase antibody or anti-endomysial antibody).

Table 3. Investigation of aphthae.

- There is a spectrum of topical anti-inflammatory agents that may help in the management of RAS.
- Topical corticosteroids can usually control symptoms. Common preparations used include four times daily:
  - Medium potency topical betamethasone sodium phosphate (eg Betnesol), or
  - Higher potency topical corticosteroids (eg beclometasone – Clenil modulite) (Table 4).

The major concern is of adrenal suppression with long-term and/or repeated application but there is no evidence that these cause this problem.

Topical tetracycline (eg doxycycline), or tetracycline plus nicotinamide may provide relief and reduce ulcer duration, but should be avoided in children under 12 who might ingest the tetracycline and develop tooth staining.

Steroid	UK trade name	Dosage every 6 hours
Medium potency Betamethasone phosphate tablets	*Betnesol*	0.5 mg ; use as mouthwash
High potency Beclometasone (Beclomethasone) dipropionate spray	*Clenil modulite*	1 puff (200 mg) to lesions

Table 4. Examples of readily available topical corticosteroids .

If RAS fails to respond to these measures, systemic immunomodulators may be required, under specialist supervision.

Keypoints for patients: aphthous ulcers

- These are common;
- They are not thought to be infectious;
- Children may inherit ulcers from parents;
- The cause is not known but some follow use of toothpaste with sodium lauryl sulphate, certain foods/drinks, or stopping smoking;
- Some vitamin or other deficiencies or conditions may predispose to ulcers;
- Ulcers can be controlled but rarely cured;
- No long-term consequences are known.

Websites and patient information

http://www.doctorsofusc.com/condition/document/11983
http://emedicine.medscape.com/article/867080-overview
http://www.cks.nhs.uk/patient_information_leaflet/mouth_ulcer

Infections

Infections that cause mouth ulcers are mainly viral, especially the herpesviruses, Coxsackie, ECHO and HIV viruses. Bacterial causes of mouth ulcers, apart from acute necrotizing ulcerative gingivitis, are less common. Syphilis and tuberculosis are uncommon but increasing, especially in people with HIV/AIDS. Fungal and protozoal causes of ulcers are also uncommon, but increasingly seen in immunocompromised persons, and travellers from the developing world.

Herpes simplex virus (HSV)

The term 'herpes' is often used loosely to refer to infections with herpes simplex virus (HSV), a ubiquitous virus which commonly produces lesions in the mouth and oropharynx. HSV is contracted by close contact with infected individuals from infected saliva or other body fluids after an incubation period of approximately 4–7 days.

Primary infection is often subclinical between the ages of 2–4 years. This is usually caused by HSV-1 and is commonly attributed to 'teething', particularly if there is a fever. However, primary infection can occur at any age and present with stomatitis (gingivostomatitis).

In teenagers or older, this may be due to HSV-2 transmitted sexually.

Generally speaking, HSV infections above the belt (oral or

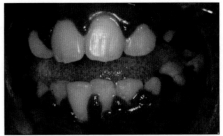

Figure 12. Primary herpetic gingivostomatitis.

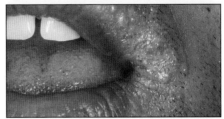

Figure 13. Herpes labialis.

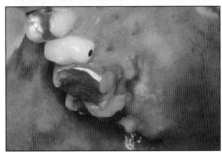

Figure 14. Lichenoid reaction to propanolol.

oropharyngeal) are caused by HSV-1 but below the belt (genital or anal) are caused by HSV-2.

The mouth or oropharynx is sore (herpetic stomatitis or gingivostomatitis): there is a single episode of oral vesicles which may be widespread, and break down to leave oral ulcers that are initially pin-point but fuse to produce irregular painful ulcers (Figure 12). Gingival oedema, erythema and ulceration are prominent and the cervical lymph nodes may be enlarged and tender, and there is sometimes fever and/or malaise. Patients with immune defects are liable to severe and/or protracted infections.

HSV is neuroinvasive and neurotoxic and infects neurones of the dorsal root and autonomic ganglia. HSV remains latent thereafter in those ganglia, usually the trigeminal ganglion, but can be re-activated to result in clinical recrudescence (see below)

Diagnosis

Diagnosis is largely clinical. Viral studies are used

occasionally and can include:
- Culture – this takes days to give a result;
- Electron microscopy – this is not always available;
- Polymerase chain reaction (PCR) detection of HSV-DNA – this is sensitive but expensive;
- Immunodetection – detection of HSV antigens is of some value.

Management

Although patients have spontaneous healing within 10–14 days, treatment is indicated particularly to reduce fever and control pain. Adequate fluid intake is important, especially in children, and antipyretics/analgesics, such as paracetamol/acetaminophen elixir, help. A soft bland diet may be needed, as the mouth can be very sore. Aciclovir orally or parenterally is useful mainly in immunocompromised patients or in the otherwise apparently healthy patient, if seen early in the course of the disease, but do not reduce the frequency of subsequent recurrences.

Recurrent HSV infections

Up to 15% of the population have recurrent HSV-1 infections, typically on the lips (herpes labialis; cold sores), from re-activation of HSV latent in the trigeminal ganglion. The virus is periodically shed into saliva, and there may be clinical recrudescence. Re-activating factors include fever such as caused by upper respiratory tract infection (hence herpes labialis is often termed 'cold' sores), sunlight, menstruation, trauma and immunosuppression.

Lip lesions at the mucocutaneous junction may be preceded by pain, burning, tingling or itching. Lesions begin as macules that rapidly become papular, then vesicular for about 48 hours, then become pustular, and finally scab within 72–96 hours and heal without scarring (Figure 13).

Recurrent intra-oral herpes in apparently healthy patients tend to affect the hard palate or gingivae with a small crop of ulcers which heals within 1–2 weeks. Lesions are usually over the greater palatine foramen, following a palatal local anaesthetic injection, presumably because of the trauma.

Recurrent intra-oral herpes in immunocompromised patients may appear as chronic, often dendritic, ulcers, often on the tongue.

Diagnosis

Diagnosis is largely clinical; viral studies are used occasionally.

Management

Most patients will have spontaneous remission within one week to 10 days, but the condition is both uncomfortable and unsightly, and thus treatment is indicated. Antivirals will achieve maximum benefit only if given early in the disease, but may be indicated in patients who have severe, widespread or persistent lesions and in the immunocompromised. Lip lesions in healthy patients may be minimized with penciclovir 1% cream or aciclovir 5% cream applied in the prodrome. In severe cases where recurrences are frequent, systemic aciclovir may be indicated. Lip lesions in immunocompromised patients require systemic aciclovir or other antivirals such as valciclovir (the precursor of penciclovir).

Keypoints for patients: cold sores

- These are common;
- They are caused by a virus (Herpes simplex) which lives in nerves forever;
- They are infectious and the virus can be transmitted by kissing;
- They may be precipitated by sun-exposure, stress, injury or immune problems;
- They have no long-term consequences;
- They may be controlled by antiviral creams or tablets, best used early on.

Websites and patient information

http://www.cks.nhs.uk/patient_information_leaflet/cold_sore
http://www.nlm.nih.gov/medlineplus/tutorials/coldsores/htm/_no_50_no_0.htm

Drug-induced ulceration

Drugs may induce ulcers by producing a local burn, or by a variety of mechanisms, such as the induction of lichenoid lesions (Figure 14). Cytotoxic drugs (eg methotrexate) commonly produce ulcers, but non-steroidal anti-inflammatory drugs (NSAIDs), including rofecoxib, alendronate (a bisphosphonate), nicorandil (a cardiac drug) and a range of other drugs, may also cause ulcers.

A drug history is important to elicit such uncommon reactions, and then the offending drug should be avoided.

Patients to refer:
- Patients with ulceration unresponsive to topical therapy;
- Malignancy;
- HIV-related ulceration;
- Syphilis;
- TB;
- Drug-related ulceration;
- Systemic disease;
- Mucocutaneous disorders.

Ulcers: Serious Ulcers

2

Malignant ulcers

A range of neoplasms may present with ulcers: most commonly these are carcinomas (Figure 1) but Kaposi sarcoma, lymphomas and other neoplasms may be seen and are discussed in Article 3. Biopsy is required to establish a definitive diagnosis.

Systemic disease

A wide range of systemic diseases, especially, mucocutaneous diseases, blood, gut and miscellaneous uncommon disorders may cause oral lesions which, because of the moisture, trauma and infection in the mouth, tend to break down to leave ulcers or erosions. Biopsy is often required to establish the diagnosis.

Mucocutaneous disorders

Mucocutaneous disease that may cause oral erosions or ulceration (or occasionally blisters) include particularly Behçet's syndrome, and a number of skin diseases including lichen planus (Figure 2), occasionally erythema multiforme or pemphigoid, and rarely pemphigus.

Behçet's syndrome

Behçet's syndrome (BS) is a rare condition. It is the association of recurrent aphthous stomatitis (RAS) with genital ulceration, and serious eye disease (especially iridocyclitis) but other systemic manifestations may also be seen. The disease is found worldwide, but most commonly in people from the Eastern Mediterranean countries (particularly Greeks, Turks, Arabs and Jews) and along the Silk route taken by Marco Polo across eastern Asia, China, Korea and Japan.

Aetiopathogenesis

Behçet's syndrome is a vasculitis which has not been proved to be infectious, contagious, or sexually transmitted. There are many immunological findings in BS similar to those seen in RAS, with T suppressor cell dysfunction, and increased polymorphonuclear leucocyte motility. There is a genetic predisposition. Many of the features of BS (erythema nodosum, arthralgia, uveitis) are common to established immune complex diseases.

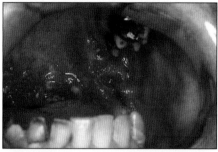

Figure 1. Squamous cell carcinoma.

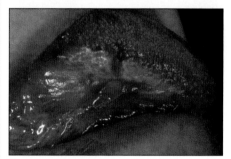

Figure 2. Lichen planus.

Clinical features

Behçet's syndrome is a chronic, sometimes life-threatening disorder characterized mainly by:
■ *Recurrent aphthous stomatitis* (RAS): in 90%–100% of cases;
■ *Recurrent painful genital ulcers* that tend to heal with scars;
■ *Ocular lesions.* Iridocyclitis, uveitis, retinal vascular changes, and optic atrophy may occur;
■ *CNS lesions;*
■ *Skin lesions*: erythema nodosum, papulopustular lesions and acneiform nodules;
■ *The joints*, epididymis, heart, intestinal tract, vascular system and most other systems may also be involved;
■ However, very non-specific signs and symptoms, which may be recurrent, may precede the onset of the mucosal membrane ulcerations by 6 months to 5 years. A history of repeated sore throats, tonsillitis, myalgias, and migratory erythralgias without overt arthritis is common.

Differential diagnosis

This is from a range of other syndromes that can affect the eyes, mouth and skin – such as various dermatological disorders and infections.

Diagnosis

BS can be very difficult to diagnose and there is no single diagnostic investigation. The International Study Group for Behçet's Disease (ISGBD) criteria suggest the diagnosis be made on clinical grounds alone on the basis of RAS plus two or more of:

- Recurrent genital ulceration;
- Eye lesions;
- Skin lesions;
- Pathergy – a >2mm diameter erythematous nodule or pustule forming 24–48 hours after sterile subcutaneous puncture of the forearm.

Investigations

There is no specific diagnostic test but typing for specific human leukocyte antigens (HLA B5101) can help. Disease *activity* may be assessed by serum levels of various proteins raised in active BS, such as the acute phase proteins (erythrocyte sedimentation rate (ESR), C-reactive protein (CRP)) or antibodies to intermediate filaments.

Management

In the face of the difficult diagnosis and serious potential complications, patients with suspected BS should be referred early for specialist advice.

Websites and patient information

http://www.arthritisresearchuk.org/arthritis_
information/arthritis_types__symptoms/behcets_
syndrome.aspx
http://www.behcets.org.uk

Lichen planus

Lichen planus is discussed in Article 6.

Erythema multiforme

Erythema multiforme (EM) is an uncommon, acute, often recurrent reaction affecting mucocutaneous tissues, seen especially in younger males.

The aetiology of erythema multiforme (EM) is unclear in most patients, but it appears to be an immunological hypersensitivity reaction, leading to sub- and intra-epithelial vesiculation.

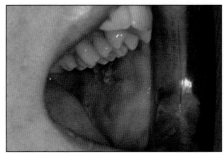

Figure 3. Erythema multiforme presenting with multiple recurrent ulcers.

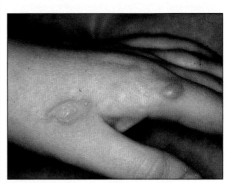

Figure 4. Erythema multiforme – skin.

There may be a genetic predisposition with associations of recurrent EM with various HLA haplotypes.

EM is triggered by a range of usually exogenous factors, such as:

- *Infective agents*, particularly HSV (herpes-associated EM: HAEM) and the bacterium *Mycoplasma pneumoniae*;
- *Drugs* such as sulfonamides (eg co-trimoxazole), cephalosporins, aminopenicillins, and many others;
- *Food additives or chemicals*.

Clinical features

EM ranges from limited disease (Minor EM) to severe, widespread life-threatening illness (Major EM). Most patients (70%) in either form, have oral lesions, which may precede lesions on other stratified squamous epithelia (eyes, genitals, or skin), or may arise in isolation. Oral EM typically presents with macules which evolve to blisters and ulcers (Figure 3). The lips become swollen, cracked, bleeding and crusted. Skin lesions start on the hands and/or feet but subsequently spread along the limbs to involve the trunk. The lesions are initially sharply demarcated macules which evolve into target-like lesions (Figure 4).

Minor EM affects only one site and may affect mouth alone, or skin, or other mucosae. Rashes are various but typically

Pemphigoid variants
Dermatitis herpetiformis
Acquired epidermolysis bullosa (EBA)
Toxic epidermal necrolysis (TEN)
Erythema multiforme
Dermatitis herpetiformis
Linear IgA disease
Chronic bullous dermatosis of childhood

Table 1. Uncommon sub-epithelial vesiculobullous disorders.

'iris' or 'target' lesions or bullae on extremities.

Major EM (Stevens-Johnson syndrome – SJS) almost invariably involves the oral mucosa and causes widespread lesions affecting mouth, eyes, pharynx, larynx, oesophagus, skin and genitals.

Diagnosis

There are no specific diagnostic tests for EM. Therefore, the diagnosis is mainly clinical, and it can be difficult to differentiate it from viral stomatitis, pemphigus, toxic epidermal necrolysis, and sub-epithelial immune blistering disorders. Serology for HSV or *Mycoplasma pneumoniae*, or other micro-organisms, and biopsy of perilesional tissue, with histological and immunostaining examination are essential if a specific diagnosis is required.

Management

Spontaneous healing can be slow – up to 2 to 3 weeks in minor EM and up to 6 weeks in major EM.

Treatment is thus indicated but controversial and thus specialist care should be sought. Supportive care is important; a liquid diet and intravenous fluid therapy may be necessary. Oral hygiene should be improved with 0.2% aqueous chlorhexidine mouthbaths.

The use of corticosteroids is controversial but minor EM may respond to topical corticosteroids. Patients with major EM, such as the Stevens-Johnson syndrome, may need to be admitted for hospital care. Major EM patients should be referred for treatment with systemic corticosteroids or other immunomodulatory drugs.

Websites and patient information

http://emedicine.medscape.com/article/1122915-overview http://www.nlm.nih.gov/medlineplus/ency/article/000851.htm

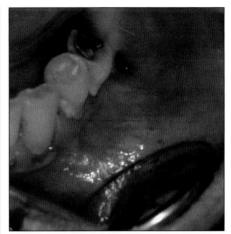
Figure 5. Pemphigoid.

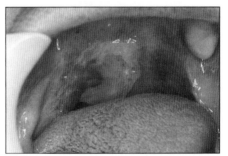
Figure 6. Mucous membrane pemphigoid.

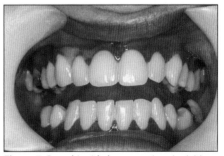
Figure 7. Pemphigoid, desquamative gingivitis.

Pemphigoid

Pemphigoid is the term given to a group of uncommon sub-epithelial immunologically-mediated vesiculobullous disorders (SEIMD) which can affect stratified squamous epithelium, characterized by damage to one of the protein constituents of the basement membrane zone (BMZ) anchoring filament components; a number of other sub-epithelial vesicullobullous disorders may produce similar clinical features (Table 1).

Variant	Oral lesions	Main antigens (Ags)	Localization Ags	Antibodies
Pemphigus vulgaris localized to mucosae (Mucosal)	Common	Dsg 3	Desmosomes	IgG
Pemphigus vulgaris also involving skin/other mucosae (Mucocutaneous)	Common	Dsg 3 Dsg 1	Desmosomes	IgG

Table 2. Main types of pemphigus involving the mouth.

The main types of pemphigoid that involve the mouth are:
■ *Mucous membrane pemphigoid* (MMP), in which mucosal lesions predominate but skin lesions are rare;
■ *Oral mucosal pemphigoid* – patients with oral lesions only, without a progressive ocular scarring process and without serologic reactivity to bullous pemphigoid (BP) antigens;
■ *Bullous pemphigoid* (BP) – which affects mainly the skin;
■ *Ocular pemphigoid* – which is sometimes termed cicatricial pemphigoid (CP) since it may cause serious conjunctival scarring.

However, most of the literature has failed to distinguish these variants, since their distinction has only recently been recognized, and therefore the following discussion groups them together.

Mucous membrane/oral pemphigoid

Mucous membrane pemphigoid (benign mucous membrane pemphigoid) is an uncommon chronic disease, twice as common in females, and presenting usually in the fifth to sixth decades.

Mucous membrane pemphigoid is an autoimmune type of disorder with a genetic predisposition. The precipitating event is unclear in most cases but rare cases are drug-induced (eg by furosemide or penicillamine).

It is characterized immunologically by deposition of IgG and C_3 antibodies directed against the epithelial basement membrane zone (BMZ). There are also circulating auto-antibodies to BMZ components, present in hemi-desmosomes or the lamina lucida.

The antibodies damage the BMZ and histologically there is a sub-basilar split. The pathogenesis probably includes complement mediated sequestration of leukocytes with resultant cytokine and leukocyte enzyme release and detachment of the basal cells from the BMZ.

Clinical features

The oral lesions (Figures 5, 6 and 7) affect especially the gingivae and palate and include bullae or vesicles which are tense, may be blood-filled and remain intact for several days. Persistent irregular erosions or ulcers appear after the blisters burst and, if on the gingivae, can produce desquamative gingivitis – the most common oral finding. This is characterized by erythematous, ulcerated, tender gingivae in a patchy, rather than continuous distribution.

The majority of people with MMP have only oral lesions but genital involvement can cause great morbidity and untreated ocular involvement can lead to blindness. Nasal, laryngeal and skin blisters are rare.

Diagnosis

The oral lesions of pemphigoid may be confused clinically with pemphigus, or occasionally erosive lichen planus, erythema multiforme or sub-epithelial blistering conditions shown in Table 1.

Biopsy of perilesional tissue, with histological and immunostaining examination can therefore be essential to the diagnosis.

Management

Spontaneous remission is rare, and thus treatment is indicated. Specialist advice is usually needed.

Systemic manifestations must be given attention. For that reason, an ophthalmology consultation is essential to rule out occult ocular disease.

The majority of cases respond well to topical corticosteroids such as are used for aphthae (Article 1). Non-steroidal immunosuppressive agents, such as tacrolimus, may be needed if the response to topical corticosteroids is inadequate.

Severe pemphigoid may need to be treated with immunosuppression using azathioprine or systemic corticosteroids.

Website and patient information

http://www.dent.ucla.edu/pic/members/MMP/

Pemphigus

Pemphigus is a group of, fortunately rare, potentially life-threatening chronic diseases characterized by epithelial blistering affecting cutaneous and/or mucosal surfaces. There are several variants with different auto-antibody profiles and clinical manifestations (Table 2) but the main type is *Pemphigus vulgaris*; this includes an uncommon variant *pemphigus vegetans*. *Pemphigus vulgaris* is seen mainly in middle- aged and elderly females of Mediterranean, Ashkenazi Jewish or South Asian descent.

Pemphigus vulgaris is an autoimmune disorder in which there is a fairly strong genetic background. Rare cases have been triggered by medications (captopril, penicillamine, rifampicin and diclofenac are the main offenders), or other factors.

The auto-antibodies are directed against stratified squamous epithelial desmosomes, particularly the proteins desmoglein-3 (Dsg3) and desmoglein-1 (Dsg1) (Table 2). Damage to the desmosomes leads to loss of cell-cell contact (acantholysis), and thus intra-epithelial vesiculation.

Clinical features

Pemphigus vulgaris typically runs a chronic course, causing blisters, erosions and ulcers on the mucosae and blisters and scabs on the skin. Oral lesions are common, may be an early manifestation, and mimic those of pemphigoid in particular. Blisters rapidly break down to leave erosions seen mainly on the palate, buccal mucosa, lips and gingiva.

Diagnosis

To differentiate pemphigus from other vesiculobullous diseases, a careful history and physical examination are important, but biopsy of perilesional tissue, with histological and immunostaining examination, are crucial. Serum should be collected for antibody titres which provides an assessment of disease activity.

Management

Before the introduction of corticosteroids, *Pemphigus vulgaris* typically was fatal, mainly from dehydration or secondary systemic infections. Specialist care is mandatory. Current treatment, by systemic immunosuppression, usually with steroids, or azathioprine or mycophenolate mofetil, has significantly reduced the mortality to about 10%.

Websites and patient information

http://www.pemphigus.org

Blood disorders that can cause ulcers include mainly the leukaemias, associated with cytotoxic therapy, viral, bacterial or fungal infection, or non-specific. Other oral features of leukaemia may include purpura, gingival bleeding, recurrent herpes labialis, and candidosis.

Gastrointestinal disease may produce soreness or mouth ulcers. A small proportion of patients with aphthae have intestinal disease, such as coeliac disease, causing malabsorption and deficiencies of haematinics, when they may also develop angular stomatitis or glossitis. Crohn's disease and *pyostomatitis vegetans* may also cause ulcers. Orofacial granulomatosis (OFG), which has many features reminiscent of Crohn's disease, may also cause ulceration.

Miscellaneous uncommon diseases such as lupus erythematosus can cause ulcers.

Differential diagnosis of oral ulceration

The most important feature of ulceration is whether the ulcer is single, multiple or persistent.
■ *Multiple non-persistent ulcers* are most commonly caused by viral infections or aphthae, when the ulcers heal spontaneously, usually within one week to one month. If this is not the case, or if the ulcers clinically do not appear to be aphthae, an alternative diagnosis such as erythema multiforme should be considered.
■ *A single ulcer that persists* may be caused by neoplasia such as carcinoma, or by chronic trauma, a chronic skin disease such as pemphigus, or a chronic infection such as syphilis, tuberculosis or a mycosis (deep fungal infection).
■ *Multiple persistent ulcers* are mainly caused by skin diseases such as lichen planus, pemphigoid or pemphigus, gastrointestinal disease, blood disease, immune defect or drugs.

In cases where the diagnosis is unclear, or where there is a single persistent ulcer, specialist referral is usually indicated.

Diagnosis of oral ulceration

Making a diagnosis of the cause for oral soreness or

Agent	Use	Comments
Benzydamine hydrochloride	Rinse or spray every 1.5 to 3 hours	Effective in reducing discomfort
Lidocaine	Topical 4% solution may ease pain	Also reduces taste sensitivity
Carboxymethylcellulose	Paste or powder used after meals to protect area	Available containing triamcinolone in Canada and the Antipodes but no longer in UK or USA

Table 3. Topical agents which may reduce pain from mucosal lesions.

ulceration is based mainly on the history and clinical features. The number, persistence, shape, character of the edge of the ulcer and the appearance of the ulcer base should also be noted. Ulcers should always be examined for induration (firmness on palpation), which may be indicative of malignancy. The cervical lymph nodes must be examined.

Unless the cause is undoubtedly local, general physical examination is also indicated, looking especially for mucocutaneous lesions, other lymphadenopathy or fever, since it is crucial to detect systemic causes such as leukaemia, or HIV infection (Figure 8).

Biopsy

Informed consent is mandatory for biopsy, particularly noting the likelihood of post-operative discomfort, and the possibility of bleeding or bruising. Care must be taken not to produce undue anxiety; some patients equate biopsy with a diagnosis of cancer. Perhaps the most difficult and important consideration is which part of the lesion should be included in the biopsy specimen.

As a general rule, the biopsy should include lesional and surrounding tissue. In the case of ulcerated mucosal lesions, most histopathological information is gleaned from the peri-lesional tissue since, by definition, most epithelium is lost from the ulcer itself. The same usually applies for skin diseases affecting the mouth, where the epithelium in the area mainly affected will, more often than not, separate, and results will be compromised. In the case of a suspected potentially malignant or malignant lesion, any red area should ideally be included in the specimen. In some cases where no obvious site can be chosen, vital staining with 'toluidine blue' may first be indicated.

A biopsy punch has the advantage that the incision is controlled, an adequate specimen is obtained (typically 4mm or 6mm diameter) and suturing may not be required.

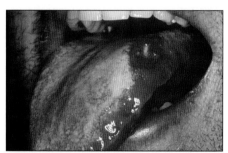
Figure 8. HIV-associated ulceration.

However, in the skin disorders, the punch can sometimes split the epithelium or detach it from the lamina propria. When a scalpel is used, a specimen of elliptical shape is usually taken, most commonly from an edge of the lesion.

Procedure

■ A local analgesic should be given although, in a few cases, conscious sedation may also be necessary.
■ Make the incisions using a scalpel with a number 15 blade.
■ Do not squeeze the specimen with forceps while trying to dissect the deep margin. A suture is best used for this purpose (and also to protect the specimen from going down the aspirator).
■ Place the biopsy specimen on to a small piece of paper before immersing in fixative, to prevent curling.
■ Put the specimen into a labelled pot, ideally in at least 10 times its own volume of buffered formalin, and leave at room temperature.
■ Suture the wound if necessary, using resorbable sutures (eg *Vicryl*).

Management of oral ulceration

■ Treat the underlying cause;

- Remove aetiological factors;
- Prescribe a chlorhexidine 0.2% mouthwash;
- Maintain good oral hygiene;
- A benzydamine mouthwash or spray or other topical agents (Table 3) may help ease discomfort.

Referral of patients with oral ulceration

Patients with single ulcers persisting more than 3 weeks, indurated ulcers, or multiple persistent ulcers may benefit from a specialist opinion.

Patients with recalcitrant ulcers, or a systemic background to mouth ulcers, or needing investigation, may also benefit from a specialist referral.

Features that might suggest a systemic background to mouth ulcers include:
- *Extra-oral features* such as skin, ocular, or genital lesions (suggestive of Behçet's syndrome); purpura, fever, lymphadenopathy, hepatomegaly, or splenomegaly (which may be found in leukaemia), chronic cough (suggestive of TB or a mycosis), gastrointestinal complaints (eg pain, altered bowel habits, blood in faeces), weakness, loss of weight or, in children, a failure to thrive.
- *An atypical history or ulcer behaviour* such as onset of ulcers in later adult life, exacerbation of ulcers, severe aphthae, or aphthae unresponsive to topical steroids.
- *Other oral lesions,* especially infections suggestive of HIV/AIDS (candidosis, herpetic lesions, necrotizing gingivitis or periodontitis, hairy leukoplakia or Kaposi's sarcoma), glossitis or angular cheilitis (suggestive of a deficiency state), or petechiae or gingival bleeding or swelling (raising the possibility of leukaemia).

Investigations which may sometimes be indicated include:
- Blood tests to exclude deficiencies, leukaemia or HIV infection;
- Microbiological and serological investigations to exclude infection;
- Biopsy;
- Immunological studies to exclude skin diseases and HIV;
- Imaging to exclude TB, deep mycoses, carcinoma, or sarcoidosis.

Patients to refer:
Patients with conditions discussed in this section should be referred for specialist care.

Ulcers: Cancer

Oral cancer

Oral cancer is the most common malignant epithelial neoplasm affecting the mouth. More than 90% is oral squamous cell carcinoma (OSCC) (Table 1).

Oral squamous cell carcinoma

Cancers of the oral cavity are classified according to site:
- Lip (International Classification of Diseases (ICD) 140);
- Tongue (ICD 141);
- Gum (ICD 143);
- Floor of the mouth (ICD 144); and
- Unspecified parts of the mouth (ICD 145).

Oral squamous cell carcinoma (OSCC) is among the ten most common cancers worldwide and seems to be increasing. The number of new mouth (oral) and

- Common
  - Squamous cell carcinoma
- Less common
  - Kaposi's sarcoma
  - Lymphomas
  - Malignant melanoma
  - Maxillary antral carcinoma (or other neoplasms)
  - Metastatic neoplasms (breast, lung, kidney, stomach, liver)
  - Neoplasms of bone and connective tissue
  - Odontogenic tumours
  - Salivary gland tumours

Table 1. Oral malignant neoplasms (with permission of CRUK).

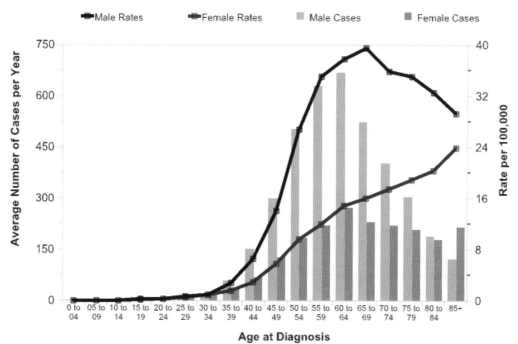

Figure 1. Oral cancer, average number of new cases per year and age-specific incidence rates, UK, 2007–2009 (with permission of CRUK).

Lesion	Aetiology	Features
Erythroplasia	Tobacco/alcohol	Flat velvet, red plaque
Leukoplakia	Tobacco/alcohol	White or speckled plaque
Actinic cheilitis	Sunlight	White plaque/erosions
Lichen planus	Idiopathic	White plaque/erosions
Submucous fibrosis	Areca nut mucosal pallor	Immobile mucosa; fibrous bands;
Discoid lupus erythematosus	Idiopathic	White plaque/erosions
Chronic candidosis	Candidal infection (most commonly *Candida albicans*)	White or speckled plaque most commonly on the buccal mucosa at the commissure
Syphilitic leukoplakia	Syphilis	White plaque
Paterson-Kelly syndrome (sideropenic dysphagia; Plummer-Vinson syndrome)	Iron deficiency	Post-cricoid web
Dyskeratosis congenita	Genetic	White plaques

Table 2. Potentially malignant oral disorders.

oropharyngeal cancers are currently estimated to be 300,000 cases world-wide, amounting to around 3% of total cancers. The mortality rate is just over 50%, despite treatment. In the UK, the total number of recorded cases of oral cancer is around 5400 per annum (Figure 1), with around 1700 deaths mainly due to late detection. The incidence appears to be rising in the UK and many other countries. In the UK, there was a 17% increase in cases of oral cancer from 3,673 (1995) to 4,304 (1999). Scotland has about double the incidence rate of oral cancer compared with England.

OSCC is seen predominantly in males but the male: female differential is decreasing. OSCC is seen predominantly in the elderly but is increasing in younger adults.

Potentially malignant states

Some potentially malignant (precancerous) *lesions* which can progress to OSCC include especially (Table 2):
■ Erythroplasia (erythroplakia; Article 7), – this is the most likely lesion to progress to carcinoma, and is very dangerous;
■ Leukoplakias (Article 6), particularly:
    – Nodular leukoplakia;
    – Speckled leukoplakia;
    – Proliferative verrucous leukoplakia;
    – Sublingual leukoplakia;
    – Candidal leukoplakia;
    – Syphilitic leukoplakia;

Some other potentially malignant (precancerous) *conditions* include:
■ Actinic cheilitis (mainly seen on the lower lip);
■ Lichen planus (mainly the non-reticular or erosive type);
■ Submucous fibrosis (mainly in users of areca nut).
■ Rarities such as:
    – Dyskeratosis congenita;
    – Discoid lupus erythematosus;
    – Paterson-Kelly syndrome (sideropenic dysphagia; Plummer-Vinson syndrome);
    – Fanconi syndrome.

Predisposing factors (risk factors)

OSCC arises because of damage to DNA (mutations) which can arise spontaneously, probably because of free radical damage, or can be caused by chemical mutagens (carcinogens), ionizing radiation or micro-organisms. OSCC arises as a consequence of multiple

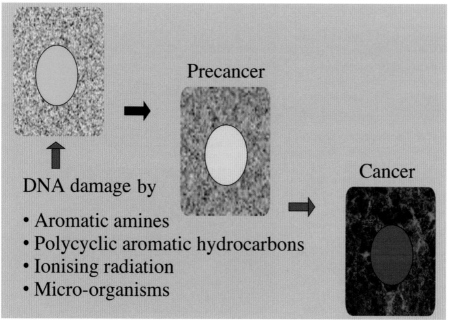

Precancer

Cancer

DNA damage by

• Aromatic amines
• Polycyclic aromatic hydrocarbons
• Ionising radiation
• Micro-organisms

Figure 2. Carcinogenesis. (Actinic radiation may predispose to lip cancer but the hazards from other types of radiation is unclear.)

molecular events causing genetic damage affecting many chromosomes and genes, and leading to DNA changes. The accumulation of genetic changes leads to cell dysregulation to the extent that growth becomes autonomous and invasive mechanisms develop – this is carcinoma (Figure 2).

Intra-oral SCC is seen especially in relation to various lifestyle habits. These are mainly tobacco and alcohol related.

Tobacco, whether smoked or chewed, releases a complex mixture of at least 50 compounds, including polycyclic aromatic hydrocarbons such as benzpyrene, nitrosamines, aldehydes and aromatic amines which are carcinogens. There is some evidence to suggest that second-hand smoke may increase oral cancer. Pipe smoking was previously associated with lip cancer. However, pipe smoking has decreased in popularity and may help explain the reduced incidence of lip cancer. The risk of oral cancer related to tobacco exposure is both duration- and dose-dependent. Smoking cessation leads to a reduction in the risk but it may take 20 years before the risk is similar to that seen in lifelong non-smokers.

Alcohol (ethanol) is metabolized to acetaldehyde, which may be carcinogenic. Nitrosamine and urethane contaminants may also be found in some alcoholic drinks. Alcohol damage to the liver might, by impairing carcinogen metabolism, also play a role.

The combination of tobacco use and alcohol consumption is particularly implicated in OSCC. People who both smoke and drink alcohol have a significantly greater risk of oral cancer than those who only smoke or drink alcohol.

Betel quid often contains betel vine leaf, betel (areca) nut, catechu, and slaked lime which, together with tobacco, appears to be carcinogenic. Some 20% of the world's population use betel. In people from the developing world, OSCC is seen especially in tobacco or alcohol users and particularly in betel quid users. Various other chewing habits, usually containing tobacco, are used in different cultures (eg Khat [Qat], Shammah, Toombak).

Other factors

All tobacco/alcohol users do not develop cancer, and similarly not all patients with cancer have these habits, and thus other factors must also play a part.
These may include:
■ *Deficiencies of vitamins* A, E or C;
■ *An impaired ability to metabolize carcinogens*; and/or
■ *An impaired ability to repair DNA* damaged by mutagens;
■ *Immune defects* may predispose to OSCC, especially lip cancer, which is increased in, eg immunosuppressed renal transplant recipients.

Clinical features

Most oral cancer is carcinoma on the lower lip where it may be preceded by, or associated with, actinic cheilitis (Figure 3) induced by chronic exposure to sunlight, and typically presents as a swelling or lump (Figure 4); the other main site is intra-orally, especially on the postero-lateral border/ventrum of the tongue (Figure 5).

Intra-oral OSCC may present as an indurated lump/ulcer, ie a firm infiltration beneath the mucosa (Figures 6 and 7); a lump sometimes with abnormal supplying blood vessels; a red lesion (erythroplasia); a granular ulcer with fissuring or raised exophytic margins; a white or mixed white and red lesion (Figure 8); a white lesion (Figure 9), a non-healing extraction socket; a lesion fixed to deeper tissues or to overlying skin or mucosa; or cervical lymph node enlargement, especially if there is hardness in a lymph node or fixation. *OSCC should be considered where any of these features persist for more than 3 weeks* (Figure 10).

It is important to note that in patients with OSCC, a *second* primary neoplasm may be seen elsewhere in the upper aerodigestive tract in up to 25% over 3 years. Indeed, many patients treated for OSCC succumb to a second primary tumour rather than a recurrence of the original tumour.

Diagnosis

Management of early cancers appears to confer survival advantage and is also associated with less morbidity and needs less mutilating surgery. Thus it is important to be suspicious of oral lesions – particularly in patients at high risk, such as older males with habits such as the use of tobacco, alcohol or betel. *There should thus be a high index of suspicion, especially of a solitary lesion.* Clinicians should be aware that single ulcers, lumps, red patches, or white patches – particularly if any of these are persisting for more than 3 weeks, may be manifestations of malignancy.

Frank tumours should be inspected and palpated to determine extent of spread; for tumours in the posterior tongue, examination under general anaesthesia by a Specialist may facilitate this.

The whole oral mucosa should be examined as there may be widespread dysplastic mucosa ('field change') or even a second neoplasm and the cervical lymph nodes and rest of the upper aerodigestive tract (mouth, nares, pharynx, larynx, oesophagus) must be examined.

Investigations

It is essential to determine whether bone or muscles are

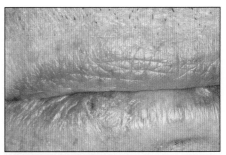
Figure 3. Actinic keratosis.

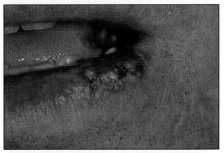
Figure 4. Early squamous carcinoma of the lip.

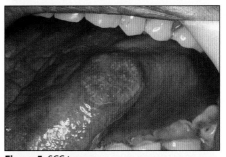
Figure 5. SCC tongue.

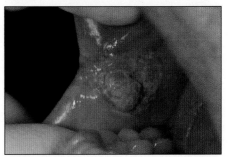
Figure 6. SCC complicating candidal leukoplakia.

involved or if metastases –initially to regional lymph nodes and later to liver, bone and brain – are present. Imaging may be needed (Figures 11 and 12). Another important aspect in planning treatment is to determine if there is malignant disease elsewhere, particularly whether other primary

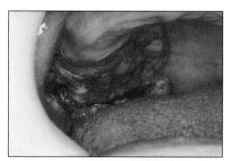

Figure 7. SCC in soft palate complex.

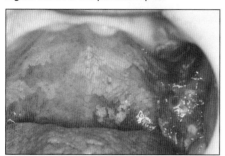

Figure 8. SCC arising in leukoplakia.

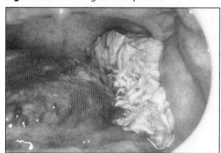

Figure 9. Squamous cell carcinoma.

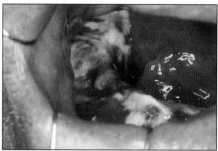

Figure 11. Squamous cell carcinoma.

tumours are present, and therefore endoscopy may form part of the initial assessment.

Urgent referral should be made but, if a Specialist opinion is not readily accessible, an incisional biopsy can be done in general practice if the practitioner is both competent and confident to carry this out. If you ARE concerned, phone, e-mail or write for an URGENT Specialist opinion, which is indicated if you feel a diagnosis of cancer is seriously possible or if the diagnosis is unclear. One of the most difficult clinical situations in which clinicians find themselves is with the patient in whom cancer is suspected. Patient communication and information are important. If the patient is to be referred to a Specialist for a diagnosis and insists (rightly) on a full explanation as to why there is a need for a second opinion, it is probably better to say that you are trained more to be suspicious but hope the lesion is nothing to worry about, though you would be failing in your duty if you did not ask for a second opinion. However, you should leave discussion of actual diagnosis, treatment

WARNING FEATURES

- Mouth sore or ulcer that does not heal
- Unexplained mouth lump or overgrowth of tissue
- White or red patches
- Difficulty in swallowing
- Unexplained difficulty in chewing, moving the jaw or tongue
- Unexplained altered sensation
- Feeling that something is caught in the throat

- Chronic sore throat or hoarseness, particularly in smokers over 50 years old and heavy drinkers
- Swelling of the jaw that causes dentures to fit poorly or become uncomfortable
- Neck swelling
- Unexplained tooth mobility
- Unilateral nasal mass, ulceration or obstruction, particularly associated with purulent or bloody discharge

Figure 10. Warning features suggestive of carcinoma.

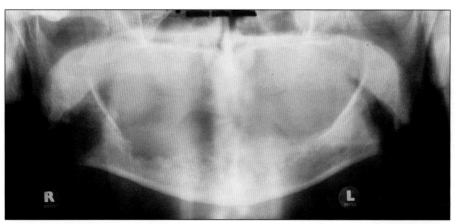

Figure 12. Radiograph from patient in Figure 11, showing bony destruction.

and prognosis to the Specialist concerned, as only he/she is in a position to give accurate facts regarding future management to the patient concerned.

The biopsy should be sufficiently large to include enough suspect tissue to give the pathologist a chance to make a diagnosis and not to have to request a further specimen. Since red rather than white areas are most likely to show dysplasia, a biopsy should be taken of the former. Some authorities always take several biopsies at the first visit in order to avoid the delay and aggravation resulting from a negative pathology report in a patient who is strongly suspected as suffering from a malignant neoplasm. Attempts to highlight clinically probably dysplastic areas before biopsy, eg by the use of toluidine blue dye and other vital stains, may be of some help where there is widespread 'field change'. Molecular techniques are being introduced for prognostication in potentially malignant lesions and tumours, and to identify nodal metastases.

Finally, the Specialist also needs to ensure that the patient is as prepared as possible for the major surgery required, particularly in terms of general anaesthesia, potential blood loss and ability to metabolize drugs, and to address any potential medical, dental or oral problems pre-operatively, to avoid complications.

Therefore, almost invariably, the following are indicated:
- Medical examination;
- Biopsy of equivocal neck lymph nodes;
- Jaw and chest radiography;
- MRI or CT;
- Electrocardiography;
- Blood tests.

Selected patients may also need:

- Bronchoscopy – if chest radiography reveals lesions;
- Endoscopy – if there is a history of tobacco use;
- Gastroscopy – if PEG (per-endoscopic gastrostomy) is to be used for feeding post-surgery;
- Liver ultrasound – to exclude metastases;
- Doppler duplex flow studies and angiography: to help in planning free flaps for reconstruction.

Management

Cancer treatment involves a team approach including a range of specialties involving surgeons, anaesthetists, oncologists, nursing staff, dental staff, nutritionists, speech therapists and physiotherapists, and others. Increasingly, Head and Neck Tumour Boards are being developed along with Cancer Networks to facilitate the collaboration of providers of cancer services to provide seamless care based on best practice. Consensus guidelines to treatment are now being published.

OSCC is now treated largely by surgery and/or radiotherapy to control the primary tumour and metastases in cervical lymph nodes. Treatment and prognosis depend on the TNM classification (Tables 3 and 4).

The planning phase includes discussions regarding restorative and surgical interventions required before cancer treatment, including osseo-integrated implants and jaw and occlusal reconstruction, and therapy is also planned to avoid post-operative complications. As much oral care as possible should be completed before starting cancer treatment.

Oral care is especially important when radiotherapy is to be given, since there is a liability particularly to

Primary tumour size (T)	
Tx	No available information
T0	No evidence of primary tumour
Tis	Only carcinoma *in situ*
T1, T2, T3, T4	Increasing size of tumour. T1 maximum diameter of 2cm; T2 maximum diameter of 4cm; T3 maximum diameter over 4cm. T4 massive tumour greater than 4cm diameter, with involvement of antrum, pterygoid muscles, base of tongue or skin
Regional lymph node involvement (N)	
Nx	Nodes could not be or were not assessed
N0	No clinically positive nodes
N1	Single clinically positive ipsilateral node less than 3cm in diameter
N2	Single clinically positive ipsilateral node 3cm to 6cm in diameter, or multiple clinically positive homolateral nodes, none more than 6cm in diameter
N2a	Single clinically positive ipsilateral node 3cm to 6cm in diameter
N2b	Multiple clinically positive ipsilateral nodes, none more than 6cm in diameter
N3	Massive ipsilateral node(s), bilateral nodes, or contralateral node(s)
N3a	Clinically positive ipsilateral node(s), one more than 6cm in diameter
N3b	Bilateral clinically positive nodes
N3c	Contralateral clinically positive node(s)
Involvement by distant metastases(M)	
Mx	Distant metastasis was not assessed
M0	No evidence of distant metastasis
M1, M2, M3	Distant metastasis is present. Increasing degrees of metastatic involvement, including distant nodes

Table 3. TNM classification of malignant neoplasms. Several other classifications are available, eg STNM (S = site).

Stage	TNM	Approximate % survival at 5 years
I	T1 N0 M0	85
II	T2 N0 M0	65
III	T3 N0 M0	40
	T1, T2 or T3 N1 M0	
IV	Any T4, N2, N3 or M1	10

Table 4. Prognosis for intra-oral carcinoma. Adapted from Sciubba JJ. Oral cancer. The importance of early diagnosis and treatment. *Am J Clin Dermatol* 2001; **2** (4): 239–251.

mucositis, xerostomia and other complications, and a risk of osteonecrosis – the initiating factor for which is often trauma, such as tooth extraction, or ulceration from an appliance, or oral infection.

Websites and patient information

http://www.mayoclinic.com/health/mouth-cancer/DS01089
http://www.oncolink.org

http://www.oralcancer.org
http://www.nlm.nih.gov/medlineplus/oralcancer.html
http://www.dh.gov.uk/PolicyAndGuidance/HealthAndSocialCareTopics/Cancer/fs/en
http://www.rdoc.org.uk/

Patients to refer:
■ All patients with suspected oral malignancy.
■ Patients with potentially malignant lesions.

Ulcers: Dry Mouth and Disorders of Salivation

4

Saliva is essential to oral health. The most obvious and important function of saliva is in eating, for taste and to lubricate food, as well as protecting the mucosa and teeth (Table 1). The water, mucins and proline-rich glycoproteins lubricate food and help swallowing. Importantly, saliva is essential for normal taste perception. Saliva is protective *via* the washing action, *via* various antimicrobial components such as mucin, histatins, lysozyme and lactoferrin, and *via* specific antibodies to a range of micro-organisms that the host has encountered.

Salivary gland secretion from the major (parotid, submandibular and sublingual) and minor glands (multiple mucous glands scattered throughout the mouth – especially the lips and soft palate), is mainly under neural control, under the influence of the autonomic nervous system, although various hormones may also modulate its composition. In general, parasympathetic stimulation increases salivation, while sympathetic stimulation produces more viscous saliva and therefore appears to depress salivation.

Thus, in acute anxiety, when there is sympathetic stimulation, the mouth feels dry. The mouth is also dry if the parasympathetic system is inhibited by, for example, various drugs. Anything that damages the glands, or reduces body fluids, can also reduce salivation.

Dry mouth (xerostomia)

Dry mouth (xerostomia) is a complaint that is the most common salivary problem and is the subjective sense of dryness which may be due to:
■ Reduced salivary flow (hyposalivation); and/or
■ Changed salivary composition.

Patients who have chronically decreased salivary flow (hyposalivation) suffer from lack of oral lubrication, affecting many functions, and they may complain of dryness (xerostomia), and can develop dental caries and other infections (candidosis, or acute bacterial sialadenitis) as a consequence of the reduced defences.

Causes

There are physiological causes of hyposalivation. Thus a

■ Digestion
■ Lubrication
■ Buffering
■ Mineralization
■ Tissue coating
■ Anti-microbial

Table 1. Functions of saliva.

■   Iatrogenic
– Drugs
– Irradiation
– Graft versus host disease
■   Disease
– Dehydration
– Psychogenic
– Salivary gland disease
– Sjögren's syndrome
– Sarcoidosis
– Salivary aplasia
■   Drugs

Table 2. Causes of dry mouth.

dry mouth is common during periods of anxiety, due to sympathetic activity; mouthbreathers may also have a dry mouth and advancing age is associated with dry mouth, probably because of a reduction of salivary acini, with a fall in salivary secretory reserve.

Very rarely, salivary glands may be absent at birth – so-called salivary gland aplasia or agenesis.

Most salivary gland dysfunction is acquired (Table 2).

In most older people complaining of xerostomia, the cause is usually due to medication or disease. Indeed, the main causes of dry mouth are iatrogenic, particularly drug use. There is usually a fairly close temporal relationship between starting the drug treatment or increasing the dose, and

- ■ **Drugs which directly damage the salivary glands**
  - ■ Cytotoxic drugs
- ■ **Drugs with anticholinergic activity**
  - ■ Anticholinergic agents such as atropine, atropinics and hyoscine
  - ■ Antireflux agents eg proton-pump inhibitors (such as omeprazole)
  - ■ Psychoactive agents with anticholinergic activities such as:
    - – Antidepressants, including tricyclic (eg amitriptyline, nortriptyline, clomipramine and dothiepin [dosulepin]), selective serotonin re-uptake inhibitors (eg fluoxetine), lithium and others
  - ■ Phenothiazines
  - ■ Benzodiazepines
  - ■ Opioids
  - ■ Antihistamines
  - ■ Bupropion
- ■ **Drugs acting on sympathetic system**
  - ■ Drugs with sympathomimetics activity eg ephedrine
  - ■ Antihypertensives; alpha 1 antagonists (eg terazosin and prazosin) and alpha 2 agonists (eg clonidine) may reduce salivary flow. Beta blockers (eg atenolol, propranolol) also change salivary protein levels.
- ■ **Drugs which deplete fluid**
  - ■ Diuretics

Table 3. Drugs associated with dry mouth.

experiencing the dry mouth. However, the cause for which the drug is being taken may also be important. For example, patients with anxiety or depressive conditions may complain of dry mouth even in the absence of drug therapy (or evidence of reduced salivary flow).

Drugs recognized as causes of reduced salivation include mainly those with anticholinergic, or sympathomimetic, or diuretic activity. These include those cited in Table 3.

Irradiation for malignant tumours in the head and neck region, such as oral cancer, can produce profound xerostomia. Other sources of irradiation, such as radioactive iodine (^{131}I) used for treating thyroid disease, may also damage the salivary glands, which take up the radioactive iodine.

Dehydration, as in diabetes mellitus, chronic renal failure, hyperparathyroidism or any fever and diabetes insipidus is an occasional cause of xerostomia.

Diseases of salivary glands can also cause salivary dysfunction. These are mainly Sjögren's syndrome (a multisystem condition discussed below); sarcoidosis; HIV disease; liver diseases; and cystic fibrosis (mucoviscidosis) (Figure 1).

Finally, it is important to recognize also that some patients complaining of a dry mouth have no evidence of a reduced salivary flow or a salivary disorder (ie they have xerostomia but not hyposalivation), and in these there may be a psychogenic reason for the complaint.

Clinical features

The patient with hyposalivation may have difficulty in:
- ■ Swallowing – especially dry foods such as biscuits (the cracker sign);
- ■ Controlling dentures;
- ■ Speaking, as the tongue tends to stick to the palate – leading to 'clicking' speech.

Patients may also complain of unpleasant taste or loss of sense of taste, or halitosis.

The patient with hyposalivation may complain of a dry mouth or these sequelae alone, or also complain of dryness of the eyes and other mucosae (nasal, laryngeal, genital). Those with eye complaints have blurring, light intolerance, burning, itching or grittiness, and sometimes an inability to cry.

Systemic features (such as joint pains) may be suggestive of

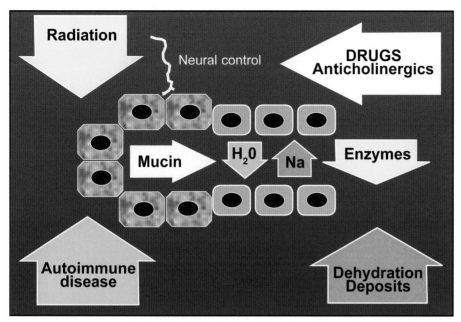

Figure 1. Causes of dry mouth. (Reproduced from Scully C. *Oral and Maxillofacial Medicine*. Elsevier, 2008.)

Sjögren's syndrome.

Examination may reveal that the lips adhere one to another, and an examining dental mirror may stick to the mucosa because of the reduced lubrication. Lipstick or food debris may be seen sticking to the teeth or soft tissues, and the usual pooling of saliva in the floor of the mouth may be absent. Thin lines of frothy saliva may form along lines of contact of the oral soft tissues, on the tongue, or in the vestibule. Saliva may not be expressible from the parotid ducts. The tongue is dry (Figure 2) and may become characteristically lobulated and usually red, with partial or complete depapillation (Figure 3).

Complications of hyposalivation can include:
■ Dental caries – which tends to involve smooth surfaces and areas otherwise not very prone to caries – such as the lower incisor region and roots (Figure 4).

Hyposalivation may explain why patients, who are apparently complying with dietary advice, have uncontrollable recurrent caries.
■ Candidosis – which may cause a burning sensation or mucosal erythema (Figure 5), lingual filiform papillae atrophy, and angular stomatitis (angular cheilitis).
■ Halitosis (Article 5).
■ Ascending (suppurative) sialadenitis – which presents with pain and swelling of a major salivary gland, and sometimes purulent discharge from the duct.

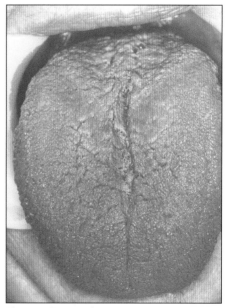

Figure 2. Dry mouth.

Diagnosis

Hyposalivation is a clinical diagnosis which can be made by the practitioner predominantly on the basis of the history and examination.

It can be helpful to document salivary function by salivary function studies, such as salivary flow rates (sialometry). Collection of whole saliva (oral fluid) is currently the routine technique for sialometry used by many clinicians, despite the fact that it is rather inaccurate and non-specific. It is usually carried out by allowing the patient to sit quietly and dribble into a measuring container over 15 minutes; in a normal person, such an unstimulated whole saliva flow rate exceeds 1.5 ml/15 min (0.1 ml/min).

Keypoints: dry mouth

Diagnosis is clinical but investigations *may* be indicated, including:
■ Blood tests (ESR and SS-A and SS-B antibodies; see below);
■ Eye tests (Schirmer; see below);
■ Urinalysis;
■ Salivary flow rate tests (sialometry);
■ Salivary gland biopsy (labial gland biopsy);
■ Imaging;
      - Sialography;
      - Scintiscanning;
      - Ultrasound;
      - Chest radiograph (if suspected sarcoidosis).

The Specialist may be needed to:
■ Study and document the degree of salivary dysfunction;
■ Determine the cause;
■ Arrange future dental care, although much of this can be undertaken in the primary care environment.

Investigations that may be indicated to exclude systemic disease, particularly to exclude:
■ Sjögren's syndrome and connective tissue disorders;
■ Diabetes;
■ Sarcoidosis;
■ Viral infections (hepatitis C; HIV).

Commonly used investigations may thus include:
■ *Blood tests* (mainly to exclude diabetes, Sjögren's syndrome, sarcoidosis, hepatitis and other infections);
■ *Eye tests* (eg Schirmer test mainly to exclude Sjögren's syndrome);
■ *Salivary gland biopsy* (if there is suspicion of organic disease, such as Sjögren's syndrome);
■ *Imaging* (mainly to exclude Sjögren's syndrome, sarcoidosis or neoplasia).

It is important to remember, as stated above that, in some patients complaining of a dry mouth, no evidence of a reduced salivary flow or a salivary disorder can be found. There may then be a psychogenic reason for the complaint.

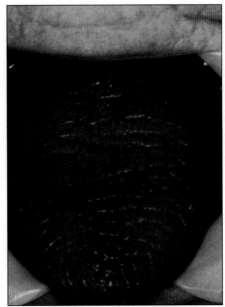

Figure 3. Xerostomia and lobulated tongue.

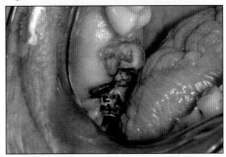

Figure 4. Dry mouth and caries in Sjögren's syndrome.

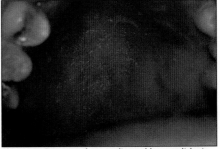

Figure 5. Dry mouth complicated by candidosis.

Management (see below)
Sjögren's syndrome

Sjögren's syndrome (SS) is an uncommon condition found

	SS-1	SS-2
Dry mouth	Yes	Yes
Dry eyes	Yes	Yes
Connective tissue disease	No	Yes
Extraglandular problems	More common	Less common

Table 4. Sjögren's syndrome.

in association with dry mouth and dry eyes. The other key features of SS are evidence of an auto-immune reaction, shown usually by serum auto-antibodies and sometimes confirmed by demonstrating mononuclear cell infiltrates in a labial salivary gland biopsy. Sjögren's syndrome can affect any age, but the onset is most common in middle age or older. The majority of patients are women with a female:male ratio of 9:1

Aetiopathogenesis

Sjögren's syndrome is an auto-immune disease affecting mainly exocrine glands like the salivary glands, lacrimal glands and pancreas. There may be a viral aetiology and a genetic predisposition.

The most common type of SS is *secondary* Sjögren's syndrome (SS-2), which comprises dry eyes and dry mouth and a connective tissue or auto-immune disease, most commonly rheumatoid arthritis (RA). Other connective tissue disorders may be associated, eg systemic lupus erythematosus and scleroderma (Table 4). However, SS can appear by itself, and in the absence of a connective tissue disease is often termed sicca syndrome, usually referred to as *primary* Sjögren's syndrome (SS-1). Nevertheless, both forms are chronic and can affect not only the salivary glands, but also extraglandular tissues. Chronic B lymphocyte stimulation can occasionally lead to B cell neoplasms, such as lymphoma.

Sjögren's syndrome is often characterized by a raised erythrocyte sedimentation rate (ESR) and several auto-antibodies – particularly antinuclear factor (ANF) and rheumatoid factor (RF), and more specific antinuclear antibodies known as SS-A (Ro) and SS-B (La).

Clinical feature

Sjögren's syndrome presents mainly with eye complaints which include sensations of grittiness, soreness, itching, dryness, blurred vision or light intolerance. The eyes may be red with inflammation of the conjunctivae and soft crusts at the angles (keratoconjunctivitis sicca). The lacrimal glands may swell.

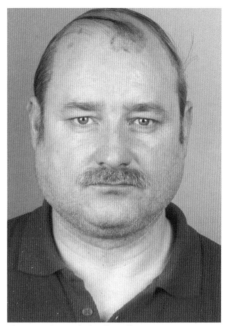

Figure 6. Parotid gland swelling.

Oral complaints (often the presenting feature) including:
■ Xerostomia;
■ Swollen salivary glands (Figure 6); causes include chronic sialadenitis as part of the fundamental auto-immune disease process, ascending bacterial sialadenitis which can arise if bacteria ascend the ducts because salivation is impaired, benign lymphoepithelial lesions/myoepithelial sialadenitis (pseudolymphoma) and lymphoma.

However, SS is a more generalized disorder which involves not only the exocrine salivary and lacrimal glands, but can have a range of other complications, summarized in Figure 7.

Diagnosis

Diagnosis is made from the history and clinical features,

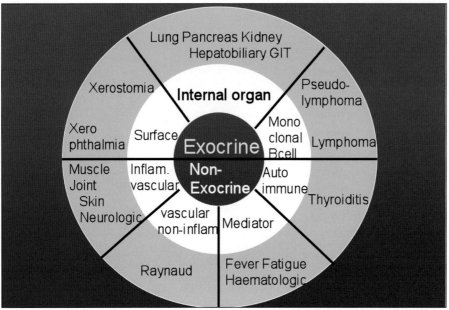

Figure 7. Sjögren's syndrome – a multisystem disease. (Reproduced from Scully C. *Oral and Maxillofacial Medicine*. Elsevier, 2008.)

and may be confirmed by auto-antibody studies and sometimes by other investigations, such as ultrasound (Figures 8 and 9), sialometry and labial salivary gland biopsy. In Specialist units various international criteria (American/European consensus diagnostic criteria) are used to confirm the diagnosis.

Management of hyposalivation

There is no specific treatment yet for SS, but the hyposalivation can be managed, and dental preventive care is essential. The dental team have an important role to play in this.

Any underlying cause of xerostomia should, if possible, be rectified; for example, xerostomia-producing drugs may be changed for an alternative, and causes such as diabetes should be treated.

Patients should be educated into efforts to avoid factors that may increase dryness, and to keep the mouth moist (Table 5).

Salivary substitutes or mouth-wetting agents may help symptomatically; various are available including:
■ Water or ice chips: frequent sips of water are generally effective;
■ Synthetic salivary substitutes (Table 6).

As patients with objective xerostomia are at increased risk of developing caries, it is important that they take a

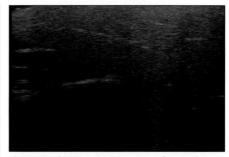

Figure 8. Ultrasound appearance of normal parotid gland showing a uniform echotexture.

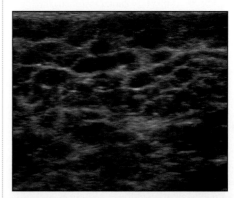

Figure 9. Ultrasound of a parotid gland showing classical appearance of Sjögren's syndrome. Multiple rounded hypo-echoic areas distributed throughout the gland.

- **Drink enough water, and sip on water and other non-sugary fluids throughout the day.** Rinse with water after meals. Keep water at your bedside.
- **Replace missing saliva** with salivary substitutes (eg *Artificial Saliva, Glandosane, Luborant, Biotene Oralbalance, AS Saliva Orthana, Salivace, Saliveze*).
  Alcohol-free mouthrinses (*BioXtra and Biotène*), or moisturizing gels (*Oralbalance, BioXtra*) may help.
- **Stimulate saliva** with:
  - Sugar-free chewing gums (eg *EnDeKay, Orbit, Biotène dry mouth gum* or *BioXtra chewing gum*); or
  - Diabetic sweets; or
  - *Salivix* or *SST* if advised; or
  - Drugs that stimulate salivation (eg pilocarpine [*Salagen*]) *if advised by a Specialist.*
- **Always take water or non-alcoholic drinks with meals and avoid dry or hard crunchy foods such as biscuits, or dunk in liquids.** Take small bites and eat slowly. Eat soft creamy foods (casseroles, soups), or cool foods with a high liquid content – melon, grapes or ice cream. Moisten foods with gravies, sauces, extra oil, margarine, salad dressings, sour cream, mayonnaise or yoghurt. Pineapple has an enzyme that helps clean the mouth. Avoid spices.
- **Avoid anything that may worsen dryness,** such as:
  - Drugs, unless they are essential (eg antidepressants);
  - Alcohol (including in mouthwashes);
  - Smoking;
  - Caffeine (coffee, some soft drinks such as Colas);
  - Mouthbreathing.
- **Protect against dental caries** by avoiding sugary foods/drinks and by:
  - Reducing sugar intake (avoid snacking and eating last thing at night);
  - Avoiding sticky foods such as toffee;
  - Keeping your mouth very clean (twice daily toothbrushing and flossing);
  - Using a fluoride toothpaste;
  - Using fluoride gels or mouthwashes (0.05% fluoride) daily before going to bed;
  - Using amorphous calcium phosphate (*Tooth Mousse*);
  - Having regular dental checks.
- **Protect against thrush, gum problems and halitosis** by:
  - Keeping your mouth very clean;
  - Keeping your mouth as moist as possible;
  - Rinsing twice daily with chlorhexidine (eg *Chlorohex, Corsodyl, Eludril*) or triclosan (eg *Plax*);
  - Brushing or scraping your tongue;
  - Keeping dentures out at night;
  - Disinfect dentures in hypochlorite (eg *Milton, Dentural*);
  - Use antifungals if recommended by Specialist.
- **Protect the lips** with a lip salve or petroleum jelly (eg *Vaseline*).
- **Avoid hot dry environments**
  - Consider a humidifier for the bedroom.

Table 5. Nine steps for managing a dry mouth.

UK trade names	Offered as	Contains fluoride	Main constituents	Comments
AS Saliva Orthana	Spray or lozenge	+/-	Mucin Xylitol	Spray contains fluoride but is unsuitable if there are religious objections to porcine mucin
Biotene Oralbalance	Gel	-	Glycerate polymer base, lactoperoxidase, glucose oxidase, xylitol	
BioXtra	Gel	-	Colostrum, lactoperoxidase, glucose oxidase, xylitol	
Luborant	Spray	+	Carboxymethylcellulose	
Glandosane	Spray	-	Carboxymethylcellulose	'Glandosane' has a low pH and therefore is best avoided in patients with a natural dentition
Saliveze				
Xerotin				
Salinum	Liquid	-	Linseed and phosphate buffer	

Table 6. Some salivary replacements (mouth-wetting agents).

non-cariogenic diet and maintain a high standard of oral hygiene. The regular use of topical fluoride agents and ACP (amorphous calcium phosphate) form important components of long-term care.

Salivation may be stimulated by using diabetic sweets or chewing gums (containing sorbitol or xylitol, not sucrose). Cholinergic drugs that stimulate salivation (sialogogues), such as pilocarpine or cevimeline, should be used only by a Specialist. Oral complications should be prevented and treated.

Keypoints for patients: dry mouth

■ Saliva helps swallowing, talking and taste, and protects the mouth;

■ Where saliva is reduced, there is a risk of dental decay (caries), halitosis, altered taste, mouth soreness and infections;

■ Saliva may be reduced by radiotherapy or chemotherapy, various drugs, after bone marrow transplant, in diabetes, in some viral infections, in anxiety/stress/depression, or in salivary gland disorders;

■ Diagnosis is clinical but investigations *may* be indicated, including:

- Blood tests;
- Eye tests;
- Urinalysis;
- Salivary flow rate;
- Salivary gland biopsy;
- X-rays or scans.

Useful websites:
http://www.bssa.uk.net/
http://www.nidcr.nih.gov/AtoZ/LetterS/
SjogrenSyndrome/
http://sjsworld.org/
http://www.nidcr.nih.gov/OralHealth/Topics/
DryMouth/

Sialorrhoea (hypersalivation; ptyalism)

Infants frequently drool but this is normal. The complaint of sialorrhoea (excess salivation) is uncommon and may be true salivary hypersecretion: usually caused by physiological factors such as menstruation or early pregnancy, local factors such as teething or oral inflammatory lesions, food or medications (those with cholinergic activity such as pilocarpine, tetrabenazine, clozapine), or bynasogastric intubation. In some cases, apparent hypersalivation is caused not by excess saliva production but by an inability to swallow a normal amount of saliva (*False sialorrhoea*) caused by neuromuscular dysfunction (eg in Parkinson's disease, cerebral palsy, or learning disability) or by pharyngeal or oesophageal obstruction, such as by a neoplasm.

Treatment is of the underlying cause if possible and then the use of behavioural approaches or antisialogogues. Occasionally, surgery to redirect the salivary gland ducts into the oropharynx may be helpful.

Patients to refer:
■ Suspected Sjögren's syndrome.

5

Halitosis

Oral malodour

Oral malodour, or halitosis, is a common complaint in adults, though few mention it, and can have a range of causes (Table 1). With oral malodour from any cause, the patient may also complain of a bad taste.

Common causes of oral malodour

Oral malodour is common on awakening (morning breath) and then often has no special significance, being usually a consequence of low salivary flow, lack of oral cleansing during sleep as well as mouthbreathing.

This rarely has any special significance, and can be readily rectified by rinsing the mouth with fresh water, eating and tongue brushing. Hydrogen peroxide rinses will also help abolish this odour.

Oral malodour at other times is often the consequence of eating various foods such as garlic, onion or spices, foods such as cabbage, brussel sprouts, cauliflower and radish, or of habits such as smoking, or drinking alcohol. Durian is a tropical fruit which is particularly malodorous.

The cause of malodour in such cases is usually obvious and avoidance of the offending substance is the logical and best prevention.

Less common causes of oral malodour

Poor oral hygiene (Figure 1) and oral infections can be responsible for oral malodour. The micro-organisms implicated in oral malodour are predominantly Gram-negative anaerobes, which include:
- *Porphyromonas gingivalis*;
- *Prevotella intermedia*;
- *Fusobacterium nucleatum*;
- *Solobacterium moorei*;
- *Tannerella forsythia (Bacteroides forsythus)*;
- *Treponema denticola*.

Gram-positive bacteria have also been implicated since they can denude the available glycoproteins of their sugar chains, enabling the anaerobic Gram-negative proteolytic bacteria to break down the denuded proteins. The Gram negative bacteria can produce chemicals that produce malodour, which include in many instances:

■ Oral sepsis
■ Dry mouth
■ Habits: smoking, alcohol and some drugs
■ Some foods
■ Starvation
■ Systemic disease
– Diabetic ketosis
– Gastro-intestinal disease
– Hepatic failure
– Renal failure
– Respiratory disease
– Trimethylaminuria
■ Psychogenic factors

Table 1. Main causes of oral malodour.

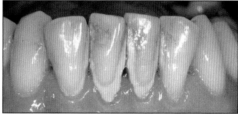

Figure 1. Oral debris, plaque, gingivitis and periodontitis are common causes of malodour.

■ Volatile sulphur compounds (VSCs), mainly methyl mercaptan, hydrogen sulphide, and dimethyl sulphide;
■ Diamines (putrescine and cadaverine);
■ Short chain fatty acids (butyric, valeric and propionic).

The evidence for the implication of other micro-organisms, such as *Helicobacter pylori*, is scant.

The posterior area of the tongue dorsum is often the location of the microbial activity associated with bad breath. Debris, such as in patients with poor oral hygiene, or under a neglected or poorly designed dental bridge or appliance, is another cause. Any patient with a dry mouth can also develop oral malodour.

Defined infective processes that can cause malodour may

include:
- Periodontal infections (especially necrotizing gingivitis (Figures 2 and 3) or periodontitis);
- Pericoronitis;
- Other types of oral infections;
- Infected extraction sockets;
- Ulcers.

Improvement of oral hygiene, prevention or treatment of infective processes, and sometimes the use of antimicrobial therapy can usually manage this type of oral malodour.

Rare causes of oral malodour

Systemic causes of oral malodour are rare but important and range from drugs to sepsis in the respiratory tract to diabetes (Table 2).

The complaint of oral malodour in the absence of malodour

The complaint of oral malodour may be made by patients who do not have it but imagine it because of psychogenic reasons. This can be a real clinical dilemma, since no evidence of oral malodour can be detected even with objective testing, and the oral malodour may then be attributable to a form of delusion or monosymptomatic hypochondriasis (self-oral malodour; halitophobia).

Other people's behaviour, or perceived behaviour, such as apparently covering the nose or averting the face, is typically misinterpreted by these patients as an indication that their breath is indeed offensive. Such patients may have latent psychosomatic illness tendencies.

Many of these patients will adopt behaviour to minimize their perceived problem, such as:
- Covering the mouth when talking;
- Avoiding or keeping a distance from other people;
- Avoiding social situations;
- Using chewing gum, mints, mouthwashes or sprays designed to reduce malodour;
- Frequent toothbrushing;
- Cleaning their tongue.

Thus the oral hygiene may be superb in such patients. Medical help may be required to manage these patients.

Such patients unfortunately fail to recognize their own psychological condition, never doubt they have oral malodour and thus are often reluctant to visit a psychology specialist.

Summary

Oral malodour can have a range of causes, though most

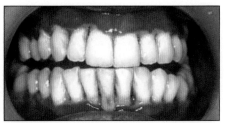

Figure 2. Acute necrotizing ulcerative gingivitis

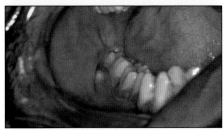

Figure 3. Necrotizing ulcerative gingivitis.

cases of true malodour have an oral cause, and many others are imagined.

Diagnosis of oral malodour

Assessment of oral malodour is usually subjective by simply smelling exhaled air (*organoleptic* method) coming from the mouth and nose and comparing the two. Odour originating in the mouth, but not detectable from the nose, is likely to be either oral or pharyngeal in origin. Odour originating in the nose may come from the sinuses or nasal passages. Children sometimes place foreign bodies in the nose, leading to sepsis and malodour! Only in the rare cases in which similar odour is equally sensed coming from both the nose and mouth can one of the many systemic causes be inferred.

Specialist centres may have the apparatus for objectively measuring the responsible volatile sulphur compounds (methyl mercaptan, hydrogen sulphide, dimethyl sulphide) – a halimeter. Microbiological investigations such as the BANA (benzoyl-arginine-naphthyl-amide) test or darkfield microscopy can also be helpful.

Keypoints: malodour (halitosis)

- Malodour is common on awakening (morning breath);
- If imagined – may signify underlying psychological problems;
- If real:
  - Is usually caused by diet, habits, dental plaque or oral disease;
  - Can be measured with a halimeter;

- Often significantly improves with oral hygiene;
- Can sometimes be caused by sinus, nose or throat conditions;
- Is *rarely* caused by more serious disease.

Management of oral malodour

The management includes first determining which cases may have an extra-oral aetiology.

A full oral examination is indicated and if an oral cause is likely or possible, management should include treatment of the cause, and other measures shown in Table 3.

In cases of malodour which may have an extra-oral aetiology, the responsibility of the general dental practitioner is to refer the patient for evaluation to a specialist. This may involve an oral medicine opinion, an otorhinolaryngologist to rule out the presence of chronic tonsillitis or chronic sinusitis, a physician to rule out gastric, hepatic, endocrine, pulmonary, or renal disease or a psychologist or psychiatrist.

Patient information and websites

http://www.tau.ac.il/~melros/

Patients to refer:
- Suspected systemic disease;
- Suspected malignancy;
- Patients with imagined halitosis.

- Drugs
  - Chloral hydrate
  - Cytotoxic drugs
  - Dimethyl sulphoxide
  - Nitrites and nitrates
  - Solvent abuse
- Respiratory problems
  - Nasal sepsis
  - Tonsillitis
  - Sinusitis
  - Lower respiratory tract infection
- Systemic disease
  - Gastrointestinal disease (some believe in an association with *Helicobacter pylori* infection)
  - Hepatic failure
  - Renal failure
  - Diabetic ketosis: the breath may smell of acetone
  - Trimethylaminuria (fish-malodour syndrome); an autosomal dominant metabolic disorder. Trimethylamine (TMA) is produced by intestinal bacteria on eating cholines (mainly in fish and eggs) and is typically oxidized by a liver enzyme. Individuals with trimethylaminuria lack this enzyme and thus secrete TMA in various bodily fluids and via their breath.
- Psychogenic factors (see below)

Table 2. Rare causes of oral malodour.

- Treat any identifiable cause (this may need antimicrobials).
- Avoid odiferous foods such as onions, garlic, spices and durian.
- Avoid habits that may worsen breath odour, such as:
  - Alcohol;
  - Tobacco.
- Eat a good breakfast, and take regular meals including fresh fruit: an enzyme in pineapple (*papain*) helps clean the mouth.
- Brush your teeth after meals.
- Keep oral hygiene regular and good:
  - Prophylaxis;
  - Toothbrushing;
  - Flossing;
  - Rinse at least twice daily with chlorhexidine (eg *Chlorohex, Corsodyl, Eludril*), triclosan (*Total*), essential oils (*Listerine*), cetylpyridinium (*MacLeans*), chlorine dioxide *(Retardex)* or other mouthwashes;
- Brush your tongue before going to bed: use a tongue scraper if that helps.
- Keep your mouth as moist as possible by using:
  - Sugar-free chewing gums (eg *Orbit, EnDeKay*);
  - Diabetic sweets.
- Use proprietary 'fresh breath' preparations eg *Dentyl pH*.
- If you have dentures, leave them out at night and in hypochlorite (eg *Dentural*) or chlorhexidine.

Table 3. Key points for patients: 10 steps towards control of oral malodour.

White Lesions

6

Truly white oral lesions appear white usually because they are keratotic (composed of thickened keratin, which looks white when wet) or may consist of collections of debris (materia alba), or necrotic epithelium (such as after a burn), or fungi (such as candidosis). These can typically be wiped off the mucosa with a gauze swab.

Other lesions, which cannot be wiped off, also appear white usually because they are composed of thickened keratin (Figure 1). A few rare conditions that are congenital, such as white sponge naevus (Figure 2), present in this way, but most white lesions are acquired and many were formerly known as 'leukoplakia', a term causing misunderstanding and confusion. The World Health Organization originally defined leukoplakia as a 'white patch or plaque that cannot be characterized clinically or pathologically as any other disease', therefore specifically excluding defined clinicopathologic entities such as candidosis, lichen planus (LP) and white sponge naevus, but still incorporating white lesions caused by friction or other trauma, and offering no comment on the presence of dysplasia. A subsequent international seminar defined leukoplakia more precisely as:

'…a whitish patch or plaque that cannot be characterized clinically or pathologically as any other disease and which is not associated with any physical or chemical causative agent except the use of tobacco.'

There is a range of causes of white lesions (Table 1), but morphological features and site may also give a guide to the diagnosis.

For example, focal lesions are often caused by keratoses; multifocal lesions are common in thrush (pseudomembranous candidosis) and in LP; striated lesions are typical of LP; and diffuse white areas are seen in the buccal mucosa in leukoedema and some LP, in the palate in stomatitis nicotina and at any site in keratoses. White lesions are usually painless but this may not be the case in burns, candidosis, LP, or lupus erythematosus.

Local causes of white lesions

Debris, burns (from heat, chemicals such as mouthwashes), grafts and scars may appear pale or white. Materia alba can usually easily be wiped off with a gauze.

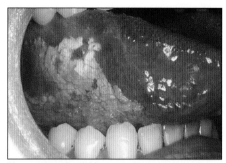

Figure 1. Leukoplakia, ventral tongue.

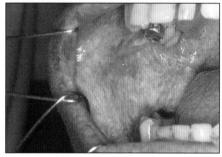

Figure 2. White sponge naevus.

Furred tongue

Tongue coating is common, particularly in edentulous adults on a soft, non-abrasive diet, people with poor oral hygiene, and those who are fasting or have febrile diseases. The coating appears more obvious in xerostomia. The coating consists of epithelial, food and microbial debris and the tongue is the main reservoir of some micro-organisms, such as Candida albicans and some Streptococci, and the various anaerobes implicated in oral malodour (Article 5).

Diagnosis

The history is important to exclude a congenital or hereditary cause of a white lesion. The clinical appearances usually strongly suggest the diagnosis: biopsy is only required if the white lesion does not scrape away from the mucosa with a gauze.

Management

Treatment is of the underlying cause where this can be identified.

Congenital causes of white lesions

Fordyce spots

Some common whitish conditions, notably Fordyce granules (ectopic sebaceous glands), are really yellowish, but may cause diagnostic confusion (Figure 3). This condition is entirely benign and does not require any further intervention, though there is some evidence they may become more prominent in hereditary nonpolyposis colorectal cancer.

Leukoedema

Leukoedema is a common benign congenital whitish-grey filmy appearance of the mucosa, seen especially in the buccal mucosae bilaterally in people of African or Asian descent. Diagnosis is clinical; the white appearance disappears if the mucosa is stretched. No treatment is available or required.

Inherited dyskeratoses

Inherited disorders of keratin are rare, but may be diagnosed, especially if there is a positive family history or other associated features, such as lesions on other mucosae, or skin appendages such as the nails.

White sponge naevus, the commonest of the inherited dyskeratoses, is an autosomal dominant condition with variable expression and a high degree of penetrance. It generally presents during childhood and is characterized by thickened, folded white patches, most commonly affecting the buccal mucosae. Other mucosal sites in the mouth may be involved and some patients may have similar lesions affecting genital and rectal mucosa. Since the other dyskeratoses may have wider implications and, in particular the risk of malignant transformation, specialist care is indicated.

Inflammatory causes of white lesions

Infections

White lesions which can result from infections include candidosis (Figure 4), hairy leukoplakia caused by Epstein-Barr virus (Figure 5), warts and papillomas (caused by human papillomaviruses) (Figure 6), and the mucous patches and leukoplakia of syphilis. Specialist care is usually indicated.

Local causes
- Materia alba and furred tongue (debris from poor oral hygiene)
- Burns
- Keratoses
  - Frictional keratosis (and cheek/lip biting)
  - Smoker's keratosis
  - Snuff-dipper's keratosis
- Skin grafts
- Scars

Congenital
- Fordyce spots
- Leukoedema
- Inherited dyskeratoses (rare, eg white sponge naevus, dyskeratosis congenita, Darier's disease)

Inflammatory
Infective
- Fungal (eg pseudomembranous and hyperplastic candidosis)
- Viral
  - Hairy leukoplakia (Epstein-Barr virus)
  - Human papillomavirus infections
- Bacterial (eg syphilitic mucous patches and keratosis)
  Non-infective
  - Lichen planus
  - Lupus erythematosus

Neoplastic and possibly pre-neoplastic
- Leukoplakia
- Keratoses
- Carcinoma

Table 1. Causes of oral white lesions.

Candidosis **(candidiasis; moniliasis)**

The importance of Candida has increased greatly, particularly as the HIV pandemic extends, since this common commensal can become opportunistic if local ecology changes, or the host immune defences fail. *Candida albicans* is the most common cause but occasionally other species may be implicated; in decreasing order of frequency these are:
- *C tropicalis*;
- *C glabrata*;

- *C parapsilosis*;
- *C krusei*;
- other Candida species and other genera.

Some 50% of the normal healthy population harbour (carry) *C albicans* as a normal oral commensal, particularly on the posterior dorsum of the tongue, and are termed Candida carriers. Candidal carriage is more common in smokers and people who wear oral appliances.

Candidosis is the state when *C albicans* causes lesions and these can be mainly white lesions (thrush particularly; Figure 4) or candidal leukoplakia (Figure 7) in which hyphal forms are common, or red lesions (denture-induced stomatitis, median rhomboid glossitis, erythematous candidosis), in which yeast forms predominate, and which may be symptomless though antibiotic stomatitis and angular cheilitis can cause soreness (Article 7).

Circumstances that cause susceptibility to candidosis include local factors influencing oral immunity or ecology, or systemic immune defects, or a combination of more than one factor (Table 2).

Diagnosis

The diagnosis of candidosis is primarily clinical but a Gram-stained smear (looking for hyphae), a microbiological swab or oral rinse for culture may help to confirm the diagnosis.

Management

Possible predisposing causes should be looked for and dealt with, if possible. Topical polyene antifungals, such as nystatin or amphotericin or imidazoles, such as miconazole or fluconazole, are often indicated.

Non-infective causes

Lichen planus (LP) is a very common cause of oral white lesions. It affects up to 2% of the adult population. Accordingly most dental practitioners will have patients afflicted with LP. It is the main skin disease that can present with oral white lesions but lupus erythematosus can present similarly. Up to 44% of patients with oral lichen planus will have skin lesions and more than 70% of patients with skin lesions will have co-incident oral lesions.

Lichen planus

Lichen planus (LP) usually affects people between the ages of 30 and 65 and there is a slight female predisposition.

Aetiopathogenesis

Lichen planus is an inflammatory autoimmune-type of

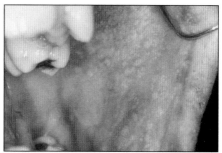

Figure 3. Fordyce spots.

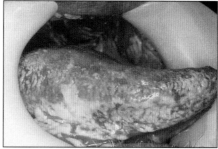

Figure 4. Pseudomembranous candidosis.

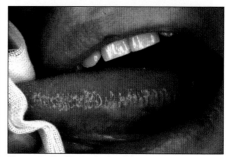

Figure 5. Oral hairy leukoplakia.

disease but it differs from classic autoimmune disorders in having no defined autoantibodies, and only rarely being associated with other autoimmune diseases. There is also no definitive immunogenetic basis yet established for LP and familial cases are rare.

Many patients afflicted with LP have a conscientious type of personality with obsessive-compulsive traits and suffer mild chronic anxiety, suggesting neuro-immunological mechanisms may be at play. Stress has been held to be important in LP: patients have a tendency to be anxious and depressed, but of course the chronic discomfort may partially explain some cases in which this association has been documented.

Pathologically, there is a local cell-mediated immunological response characterized by a dense T-lymphocyte inflammatory cell infiltrate in the upper lamina propria

Local factors influencing oral immunity or ecology	Systemic immune defects
Hyposalivation	Malnutrition
Smoking	Immunosuppressant drugs such as corticosteroids
Corticosteroids	T lymphocyte defects, especially HIV infection, leukaemias, lymphomas and cancers
Broad spectrum antimicrobials	Neutrophil leukocyte defects, such as in diabetes
Cytotoxic chemotherapy	Cytotoxic chemotherapy
Irradiation involving the mouth/salivary glands	Anaemia
Dental appliances	

Table 2. Factors predisposing to candidosis.

causing cell death (apoptosis) in the basal epithelium, probably caused by the production of cytokines such as tumour-necrosis factor alpha (TNFα) and interferon gamma (IFN-γ).

The antigen responsible for this immune response is unclear but lesions very similar to LP, termed lichenoid lesions, are sometimes caused by:
■ Dental restorative materials (mainly amalgam and gold);
■ Drugs (non-steroidal anti-inflammatory agents, antihypertensive agents, antimalarials, and many other drugs);
■ Chronic graft-versus-host disease seen in bone marrow (haemopoietic stem cell) transplant patients;
■ Infection with hepatitis C virus(in some populations such as those from southern Europe and Japan);
■ A variety of other systemic disorders such as hypertension and diabetes (probably a reaction to the drugs used).

Clinical features

Lichen planus can affect stratified squamous epithelium of the skin, the oral mucosa and genitalia.

Oral LP may present a number of different clinical pictures (Figures 8–13), including:
■ Papular LP, white papules (Figure 8);
■ Reticular LP, a network of raised white lines or striae (reticular pattern) (Figures 9, 10);
■ Plaque-like LP, simulating leukoplakia;
■ Atrophic red atrophic areas, simulating erythroplasia (Figure 11; mixed atrophic/erosive form): lichen planus is

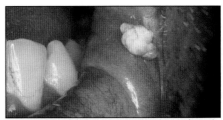
Figure 6. Condyloma acuminatum (genital wart).

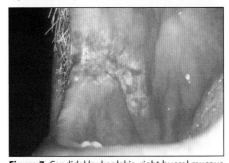
Figure 7. Candidal leukoplakia, right buccal mucous.

one of the most common causes of desquamative gingivitis;
■ Erosive erosions, less common, but persistent, irregular and painful, with a yellowish slough (Figure 12).

White lesions of LP are often asymptomatic, but there may be soreness if there are atrophic areas or erosions.

Lichen planus typically results in lesions, which are usually in the posterior buccal mucosa bilaterally, but the tongue or gingivae are other sites commonly affected.

On the skin, lichen planus frequently presents as a flat-topped purple polygonal and pruritic papular rash most often seen on the front (flexor surface) of the wrists (Figure 13) in which lesions are often crossed by fine white lines (Wickham's striae; Figure 14). Nail lesions may be seen (Figure 15). Oral LP may be accompanied by vulvovaginal lesions (the vulvovaginal-gingival syndrome).

Prognosis

Often, the onset of LP is slow, taking months to reach its peak. It usually clears from the skin within 18 months but in a few people persists for many years. Oral lesions often persist. There is no sign or test to indicate which patients will develop only oral, or oral and extra-oral lesions of LP.

Non-reticular oral LP in particular has a small malignant potential, probably of the order of 1%.

Diagnosis

LP is often fairly obviously diagnosed from the clinical features but, since it can closely simulate other conditions such as:
- Lupus erythematosus;
- Chronic ulcerative stomatitis;
- Keratosis; or even
- Carcinoma;

biopsy and histopathological examination of lesional tissue, occasionally aided by direct immunostaining, are often indicated.

Keypoints: lichen planus

- Some patients also have the condition on the skin, hair, nails or genitals;
- Diabetes, drugs, dental fillings and HCV should be excluded;
- Blood tests may therefore be required;
- Biopsy is usually in order;
- Non-reticular lichen planus *may rarely*, after years, lead to a tumour;
- Removal of the affected area does not necessarily remove the problem;
- Therefore, the best management is usually to ensure the mouth is checked by a healthcare professional at least at 6-monthly intervals.

Management

Treatment of LP is not always necessary, unless there are symptoms. Predisposing factors should be corrected:

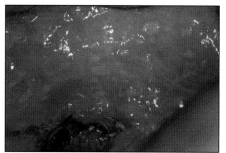
Figure 8. Papular lichen planus.

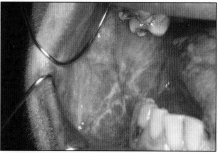
Figure 9. Reticular lichen planus.

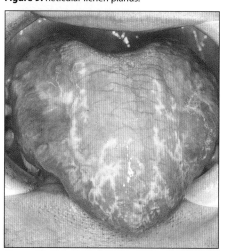
Figure 10. Reticular lichen planus, dorsum of tongue.

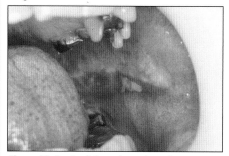
Figure 11. Erosive lichen planus, buccal mucosa.

■ It may be wise to consider removal of dental amalgams if the lesions are closely related to these, or unilateral, but tests such as patch tests will not reliably indicate which patients will benefit from this. Accordingly, empirical replacement of amalgam restorations may be indicated.

■ If drugs are implicated, the physician should be consulted as to the possibility of changing drug therapy.

■ If there is HCV infection, this should be managed by a general physician.

■ Improvement in oral hygiene may result in some subjective benefit; chlorhexidine or triclosan mouthwashes may help. Symptoms can often be controlled, usually with topical corticosteroids or sometimes with tacrolimus.

■ If there is severe or extensive oral involvement, if LP fails to respond to topical medications, or if there are extra-oral lesions, specialist referral may be indicated.

■ Patients with non-reticular lichen planus should be monitored to exclude development of carcinoma. Tobacco and alcohol use should be minimized.

Keypoints for patients: lichen planus

■ This is a common condition;
■ The cause is unknown;
■ Children do not usually inherit it from parents;
■ It is not thought to be infectious;
■ It is sometimes related to diabetes, drugs, dental fillings, or other conditions;
■ It sometimes affects the skin, hair, nails or genitals;
■ Blood tests and biopsy may be required;
■ The condition tends to persist in the mouth but it can be controlled;
■ Most lichen planus is benign but *some forms may rarely*, after years, lead to a tumour;

Therefore, the best management is usually to:
■ Avoid habits such as use of tobacco, alcohol or betel (and, for lips, sun-exposure);
■ Take a healthy diet rich in fresh fruit and vegetables;
■ Have your mouth checked by a healthcare professional at least at 6-monthly intervals;
■ Changes that might suggest a tumour is developing could include any of the following persisting more than 3 weeks:
 – A sore on the lip or in the mouth that does not heal;
 – A lump on the lip or in the mouth or throat;
 – A white or red patch on the gums, tongue, or lining of the mouth;
 – Unusual bleeding, pain, or numbness in the mouth;
 – A sore throat that does not go away, or a feeling that something is caught in the throat;
 – Difficulty or pain with chewing or swallowing;
 – Swelling of the jaw that causes dentures to fit poorly or become uncomfortable;
 – Pain in the ear;
 – Enlargement of a neck lymph gland.

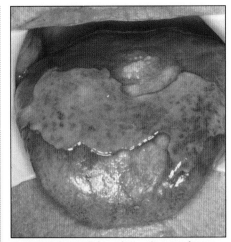
Figure 12. Erosive lichen planus, dorsum of tongue.

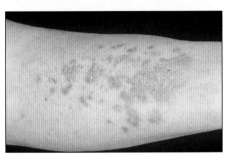
Figure 13. Lichen planus, skin.

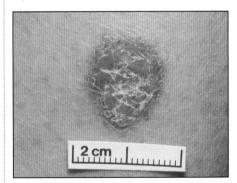
Figure 14. Cutaneous lichen planus.

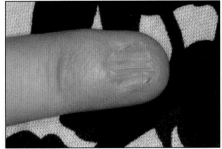
Figure 15. Nail lichen planus.

Websites and patient information

http://www.bcd.tamhsc.edu/outreach/lichen/index.
html
http://www.aad.org/pamphlets/lichen.html

Keratoses and leukoplakias

Frictional keratosis

Frictional keratosis is quite common and caused particularly by friction from the teeth and seen mainly at the occlusal line in the buccal mucosae, particularly in adult females, especially in those with temporomandibular pain-dysfunction syndrome. It is also commonly seen on the lateral borders of the tongue (Figure 16). Patients with missing teeth may develop keratosis on the alveolar ridge simply related to trauma when eating (Figure 17).

Malignant change is very rare but any sharp edges of teeth or appliances should be removed and the patient counselled about the habits.

Tobacco-induced keratoses

Tobacco is a common cause of keratosis, seen especially in males, the teeth are usually nicotine-stained and there may be mucosal smoker's melanosis but malignant change is uncommon in most forms (Table 3).

Idiopathic keratoses

Many leukoplakias are uncommon and arise in the absence of any identifiable predisposing factors and most, up to 70% in large series, are benign without any evidence of dysplasia. However, the remaining 10–30% may be, or may become, either dysplastic or invasive carcinomas. Overall, the rate of malignant transformation of all keratoses and leukoplakias is of some 3–6% over 10 years.

The lesions of greatest malignant potential are those leukoplakias which are:
■ Speckled (Figure 18), nodular (Figure 19) or verrucous lesions;
■ In at risk sites – lateral tongue, ventral tongue (Figure 20), floor of mouth (Figures 21 and 22) and soft palate complex (Figure 23);
■ Associated with *Candida* (Figure 7).

In these, rates of malignant transformation up to 30% have been reported in some series.

Diagnosis

The nature of white lesions can often only be established after further investigation.

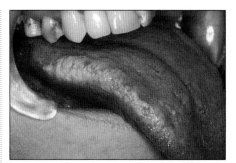

Figure 16. Frictional keratosis, lateral tongue.

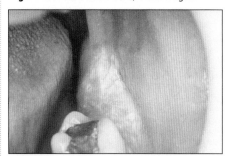

Figure 17. Frictional keratosis, retromolar pad.

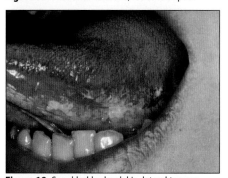

Figure 18. Speckled leukoplakia, lateral tongue.

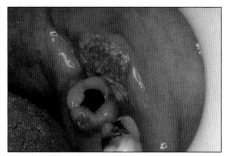

Figure 19. Nodular leukoplakia.

Biopsy is usually indicated, particularly where there is a high risk of malignant transformation, such as in lesions with:
■ Any suggestion of malignancy;
■ Admixture with red lesions (speckled leukoplakia or

Tobacco habit	Common sites affected	Occasional sites affected	Malignant potential
Cigarette	Lip (occasionally nicotine-stained) and commissures	Palate Others	Rare
Pipe smoking	Palate (termed smoker's keratosis or stomatitis nicotina)	Others	Rare
Cigar	Palate (termed smoker's keratosis or stomatitis nicotina)	Others	Rare
Snuff	Gingival (together with recession)	Lip	Rare
Reverse smoking (Bidi) *cigarettes are smoked with the lit end within the mouth*	Palate	Others	Common
Tobacco chewing	Buccal	Others	Common

Table 3. Tobacco-induced keratoses.

erythroleukoplakia);
■ A raised lesion (nodular or verrucous leukoplakia);
■ Candidal leukoplakia;
■ Floor of mouth leukoplakia (sublingual keratosis);
■ A rapid increase in size;
■ Change in colour;
■ Ulceration;
■ Pain;
■ Regional lymph node enlargement.

Keypoints: keratosis (leukoplakia)

■ Biopsy is mandatory in high risk lesions or high risk patients;
■ In a *very small* number of keratoses, and after years, a tumour may develop;
■ There is no universally agreed management;
■ Removal of the affected area does not necessarily remove the problem but does permit better histological examination.

Therefore, the best management is usually to:

■ Remove the lesion, where possible;
■ Avoid harmful habits such as use of tobacco, alcohol or betel (and, for lips, sun exposure);
■ Advise a healthy diet rich in fresh fruit and vegetables;
■ Examine the oral mucosa at least at 6-monthly intervals.

Prognosis

The finding by the pathologist of epithelial dysplasia may be predictive of malignant potential, but this is not invariable, and there can be considerable inter- and intra-examiner variation in the diagnosis of dysplasia.

Thus there has been a search for molecular markers to predict exactly which lesions are truly of malignant potential and may develop into oral squamous cell carcinoma (OSCC).

The most predictive of the molecular or cellular markers thus far assessed for OSCC development, apart from dysplasia, include chromosomal polysomy, the tumour suppressor p53 protein expression, and loss of heterozygosity (LOH) at chromosome 3p or 9p. Routine use of these is, however, hampered by their complexity and lack of facilities in many pathology laboratories.

As a surrogate for individual molecular markers, measurement of gross genomic damage (DNA ploidy) may be a realistic option, and is now available in some oral pathology laboratories.

Management

The dilemma in managing patients with potentially malignant oral lesions and field change has been deciding which mucosal lesions or areas will progress to carcinoma. At present there are no reliable markers which predict which lesions will progress. Specialist referral is indicated.

Cessation of dangerous
habits such as tobacco and/or betel use (Figures 24, 25), and the removal of lesions is probably the best course of action, particularly if they are the high risk lesions or in a high risk group for carcinoma (Article 3).
Perhaps surprisingly, management of leukoplakias is very controversial, since
there are no randomized, controlled, double-blind studies that prove the best type of treatment. However, most specialists prefer removal of the lesion (by laser, scalpel or
other means).

Keypoints for patients: keratosis (leukoplakia)

This is an uncommon condition:
■ Sometimes it is caused by friction or tobacco;
■ It is not inherited;
■ It is not known to be infectious;
■ Blood tests and biopsy may be required;
■ In a *very small* number, and after years, it may lead to a tumour;
■ There is no universally agreed management and this can be by simple observation, drugs, or surgery;

Therefore, the best management is usually to:
■ Avoid harmful habits such as use of tobacco, alcohol or betel (and, for lips, sun exposure);
■ Take a healthy diet rich in fresh fruit and vegetables;
■ Have your mouth checked by a healthcare professional at least at 6-monthly intervals;

Changes that might suggest a tumour is developing could include any of the following persisting for more than 3 weeks:

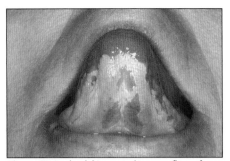

Figure 20. Leukoplakia, ventral tongue, floor of mouth.

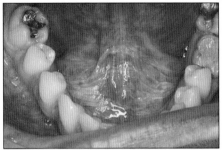

Figure 21. Leukoplakia, floor of mouth.

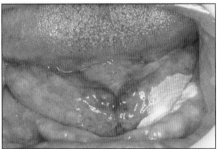

Figure 22. Sublingual leukoplakia.

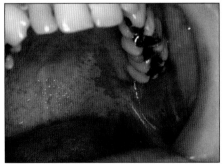

Figure 23. Leukoplakia soft palate complex.

■ A sore on the lip or in the mouth that does not heal;
■ A lump on the lip or in the mouth or throat;
■ A white or red patch on the gums, tongue, or lining of the

mouth;
- Unusual bleeding, pain, or numbness in the mouth;
- A sore throat that does not go away, or a feeling that something is caught in the throat;
- Difficulty or pain with chewing or swallowing;
- Swelling of the jaw that causes dentures to fit poorly or become uncomfortable;
- A change in the voice; and/or
- Pain in the ear;
- Enlargement of a neck lymph gland.

Useful websites and patient information

http://www.cochrane.org/cochrane/revabstr/ab001829.htm
http://www.emedicine.com/ent/topic731.htm
http://www.mayoclinic.com/health/leukoplakia/DS00458

Patients to refer:
- Keratoses which do not regress after elimination of aetiological factors;
- Hairy leukoplakia, if underlying cause of immunosuppression not already identified;
- Carcinoma.

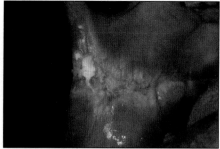

Figure 24. Betel chewing keratosis.

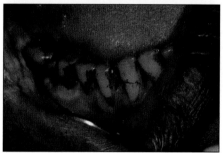

Figure 25. Same patient as Figure 23, showing tooth staining.

Red and Pigmented Lesions

7

This article covers first red lesions and then hyperpigmentation.

Red oral lesions

Red oral lesions are commonplace and usually associated with inflammation in, for example, mucosal infections. However, red lesions can also be sinister by signifying severe dysplasia in erythroplasia, or malignant neoplasms (Table 1).

Inflammatory lesions

Most red lesions are inflammatory, usually:
■ Geographic tongue (erythema migrans) (Figure 1) ;
■ Viral infections (eg herpes simplex stomatitis);
■ Fungal infections;
■ Candidosis;
 – Denture-related stomatitis; discussed below, is usually a form of mild chronic erythematous candidosis consisting of inflammation beneath a denture, orthodontic or other appliance (Figure 2);
 – Median rhomboid glossitis; a persistent red, rhomboidal depapillated area in the midline dorsum of the tongue (Figure 3);
 – Acute oral candidosis; may cause widespread erythema and soreness, sometimes with thrush, often a complication of corticosteroid or antibiotic therapy. Red lesions of candidosis may also be seen in HIV disease, typically in the palate (Figure 4);
■ Bacterial infections;
■ Cancer treatment-related mucositis; common after irradiation of tumours of the head and neck, or chemotherapy, eg for leukaemia;
■ Immunological reactions; such as lichen planus, plasma cell gingivostomatitis, granulomatous disorders (sarcoidosis, Crohn's disease, orofacial granulomatosis), amyloidosis, and graft versus host disease.

Geographic tongue (erythema migrans)

Geographic tongue (erythema migrans) is a very common condition and cause of sore tongue, affecting at least 1–2% of patients. There is a genetic background, and often

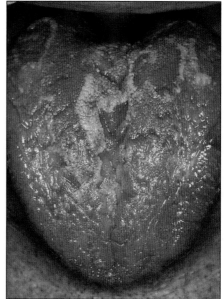

Figure 1. Geographic tongue.

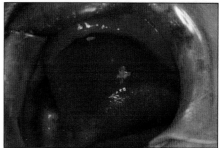

Figure 2. Candida-associated denture stomatitis.

a family history. Many patients with a fissured tongue (scrotal tongue) also have geographic tongue. Erythema migrans is associated with psoriasis in 4% and the histological appearances of both conditions are similar.

Some patients have atopic allergies, such as hay fever, and a few relate the oral lesions to various foods, eg cheese. A few have diabetes mellitus.

Clinical features

Geographic tongue typically involves the dorsum of the tongue, sometimes the ventrum and, on occasions, it may affect other oral mucosal sites. It is often asymptomatic, but a small minority of patients complain of soreness and these patients are virtually invariably middle-aged. If sore, this may be noted especially with acidic foods (eg tomatoes or citrus fruits) or cheese.

There are irregular, pink or red depapillated map-like areas, which change in shape, increase in size, and spread or move to other areas, sometimes within hours (Figure 5).

The red areas are surrounded by distinct yellowish slightly raised margins (Figure 6). There is increased thickness of the intervening filiform papillae.

Diagnosis

The diagnosis of geographic tongue is clinical mainly from the history of a migrating pattern and the characteristic clinical appearance. Blood examination may rarely be necessary to exclude diabetes, or anaemia, if there is confusion with a depapillated tongue of glossitis.

Keypoints: geographic tongue
■ The cause is unknown but it may be inherited;
■ It resembles, and is associated rarely with, psoriasis;
■ It has no long-term consequences;
■ There is no cure and treatment is therefore aimed at controlling symptoms and reassuring the patient.

Management

Reassurance remains the best that can be given. Zinc sulphate 200 mg three times daily for 3 months or a topical rinse with 7% salicylic acid in 70% alcohol are advocated by some and may occasionally help.

Keypoints for patients: geographic tongue
■ This is a common condition;
■ The cause is unknown;
■ It may be inherited;
■ There may be an allergic component;
■ It is not thought to be infectious;
■ It is associated, rarely, with psoriasis;
■ It has no long-term consequences.

Patient information and websites:

http://www.eaom.eu/files/geographic_tongue.pdf
**http://www.mayoclinic.com/health/geographic-tongue/
DS00819**

Denture-related stomatitis (denture-induced stomatitis;

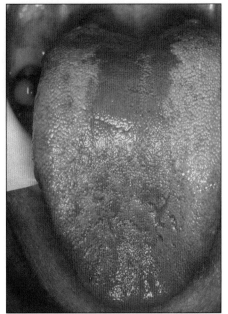

Figure 3. Median rhomboid glossitis.

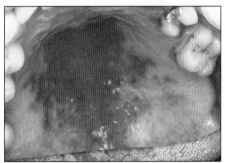

Figure 4. Erythematous candidosis.

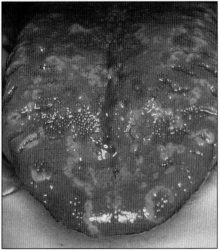

Figure 5. Geographic tongue.

denture sore mouth; chronic erythematous candidosis)

Denture-related stomatitis consists of mild inflammation of the mucosa beneath a denture – usually a complete upper denture. This is a common condition, mainly of the middle-aged or elderly; more prevalent in women than men.

Aetiopathogenesis

Dental appliances (mainly dentures), especially when worn throughout the night, or a dry mouth, favour development of this infection. It is not caused by allergy to the dental material (if it were, it would affect mucosae other than just that beneath the appliance).

However, it is still not clear why only some denture-wearers develop denture-related stomatitis, since most patients appear otherwise healthy.

Dentures can produce a number of ecological changes; the oral flora may be altered and plaque collects between the mucosal surface of the denture and the palate.

The accumulation of microbial plaque (bacteria and/ or yeasts) on, and attached to, the fitting surface of the denture and the underlying mucosa produces an inflammatory reaction. When Candida is involved, the more common terms 'candida-associated denture stomatitis', 'denture-induced candidosis' or 'chronic erythematous candidosis' are used.

In addition, the saliva that is present between the maxillary denture and the mucosa may have a lower pH than usual. Denture-related stomatitis is not exclusively associated with infection, and occasionally mechanical irritation is at play.

Clinical features

The characteristic presenting features of denture-related stomatitis are chronic erythema and oedema of the mucosa that contacts the fitting surface of the denture (Figure 2). Uncommon complications include:
■ Angular stomatitis (soreness and erythema at the commissures (Figure 7);
■ Papillary hyperplasia in the vault of the palate.

Classification

Denture-related stomatitis has been classified into three clinical types (Newton's classification), increasing in severity:
■ A localized simple inflammation or a pinpoint hyperaemia;
■ An erythematous or generalized simple type presenting as more diffuse erythema involving a part of, or the entire, denture-covered mucosa;

LOCALIZED
Inflammatory lesions
Geographic tongue
Candidosis
Lichen planus
Drug reactions
Reactive lesions
Pyogenic granulomas
Peripheral giant cell granulomas
Atrophic lesions
Geographic tongue
Lichen planus
Lupus erythematosus
Erythroplasia
Vitamin B$_{12}$ deficiency
Purpura
Trauma
Thrombocytopenia
Vascular
Telangiectases (hereditary haemorrhagic telangiectasia or scleroderma)
Angiomas (vascular hamartomas)
Neoplasms
Squamous carcinoma
Kaposi's sarcoma
Giant cell tumour
Wegener's granulomatosis
GENERALIZED
Candidosis
Avitaminosis B complex (rarely)
Irradiation or chemotherapy-induced mucositis
Polycythaemia

Table 1. Most common causes of red lesions.

■ A granular type (inflammatory papillary hyperplasia) commonly involving the central part of the hard palate and the alveolar ridge.

Diagnosis

Denture-related stomatitis and angular stomatitis are clinical diagnoses, although may be confirmed by microbiological investigations. In addition, haematological and biochemical investigations may be appropriate to identify any underlying predisposing factors, such as hyposalivation, nutritional deficiencies, anaemia and diabetes mellitus in patients unresponsive to conventional management.

Keypoints for dentists: denture-related stomatitis
■ Denture-related stomatitis is caused mainly by a yeast (Candida), but bacteria may also be involved;
■ It may be precipitated by prolonged wearing of a dental appliance, especially at night;
■ It predisposes to angular cheilitis;

It is best controlled by:
■ Leaving out the appliance, allowing the mouth to heal;
■ Disinfecting the appliance (as per additional instructions);
■ Using antifungal creams or gels (eg miconazole; *Daktarin*), oral suspension (eg nystatin; *Nystan*) or capsules (fluconazole; *Diflucan*) regularly for up to 4 weeks;
■ The appliance may require adjustment or changing;
■ Blood tests, microbiological studies or biopsy *may* be required if the lesion is unresponsive.

Management

The denture plaque and fitting surface is infested with micro-organisms, most commonly *Candida albicans* and, therefore, to prevent recurrence, dentures should be left out of the mouth at night, and stored in an appropriate antiseptic which has activity against yeasts (Table 2).

Cleansers containing alkaline hypochlorites, disinfectants, or yeast lytic enzymes are most effective against Candida. Denture soak solution containing benzoic acid is taken up into the acrylic resin and can completely eradicate *C albicans* from the denture surface. Chlorhexidine gluconate can also eliminate *C albicans* on the denture surface and a mouthwash can reduce the palatal inflammation. A protease-containing denture soak (Alcalase protease) is also an effective way of removing denture plaque, especially when combined with brushing.

The mucosal infection is eradicated by brushing the palate with chlorhexidine mouthwash or gel, and using miconazole gel, nystatin oral suspension or fluconazole, administered concurrently with an oral antiseptic, such as chlorhexidine, which has antifungal activity.

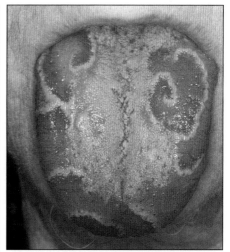

Figure 6. Geographic tongue.

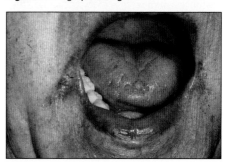

Figure 7. Angular stomatitis (cheilitis).

Denture hygiene measures
Antifungal therapy (eg topical or systemic)
If unresponsive to above, investigate for underlying predisposing factors

Table 2. Management of denture-related stomatitis.

Keypoints for patients: denture sore mouth (denture-related stomatitis)
■ Denture sore mouth is common, but rarely sore;
■ It is caused mainly by a yeast (Candida) that usually lives harmlessly in the mouth and elsewhere;
■ It is not transmitted to others;
■ It may be precipitated by prolonged wearing of a dental appliance, especially at night, which allows the yeast to grow;
■ It predisposes to sores at the corners of the mouth (angular cheilitis);
■ It has no serious long-term consequences;
■ Blood tests, microbiological studies or biopsy *may* be required.

It is best controlled by:
- Leaving out the appliance, allowing the mouth to heal;
- Cleaning the appliance (as below);
- Disinfecting the appliance (as per additional instructions);
- Using antifungal creams or gels regularly for up to 4 weeks;
- The appliance may require adjustment or changing;
- Keep the appliance as clean as natural teeth. Clean both surfaces (inside and outside) after meals and at night. Use washing-up liquid and a toothbrush and lukewarm water and hold it over a basin containing water, in case you drop it, which could cause it to break. Never use hot water, as it may alter the colour. A disclosing agent, for example *Rayners Blue* or *Red food colouring* (available at most supermarkets) can be applied with cotton buds, to help see whether you are cleaning the appliance thoroughly enough. If stains or calculus deposits are difficult to remove, try an overnight immersion (eg *Dentural, Milton* or *Steradent*), or an application of *Denclen*.

Dentures should be left out overnight, so that your mouth has a rest. It is not natural for your palate to be covered all the time and the chances of getting an infection are increased if the dentures are worn 24 hours a day. Ensure you leave the dentures out for at least some time and keep them in *Dentural* or *Steradent*, as they may distort if allowed to dry out.

Special precautions for dentures with metal parts; *Denclen, Dentural* and *Milton* may discolour metal, so use with care. Brush briefly to remove stains and deposits, rinse well with lukewarm water and do not soak overnight.

Before re-use, wash in water and brush the appliance to remove loosened deposits.

Website and patient information

http://emedicine.medscape.com/article/1075994-overview

Neoplastic lesions: red neoplasms include:
- Peripheral giant cell tumours;
- Angiosarcomas, such as Kaposi's sarcoma, a common neoplasm in HIV/AIDS, appears in the mouth as red or purplish areas or nodules, especially seen in the palate;
- Squamous cell carcinomas;
- Wegener's granulomatosis.

Vascular anomalies (angiomas and telangiectasia) include:
- Dilated lingual veins (varices) may be conspicuous in elderly persons; this is part of the normal spectrum;
- Haemangiomas (Figures 8–10) are usually small

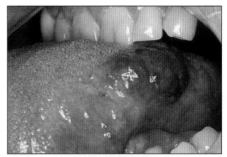

Figure 8. Vascular hamartoma (haemangioma on tongue).

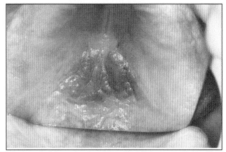

Figure 9. Vascular hamartoma (haemangioma in palate).

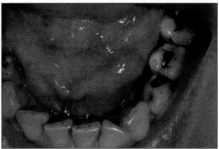

Figure 10. Haemangioma in floor of mouth.

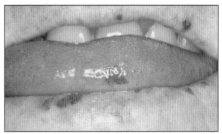

Figure 11. Telangiectasia, lips and tongue.

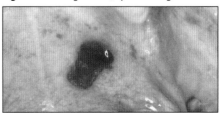

Figure 12. Angina bullosa haemorrhagica.

isolated developmental anomalies, or hamartomas;
■ Telangiectasias (Figure 11) – dilated capillaries – may be seen after irradiation and in disorders such as hereditary haemorrhagic telangiectasia and systemic sclerosis.

Angiomas are benign and usually congenital. In general, most do not require any active treatment, unless symptoms develop, in which case they can be treated by injection of sclerosing agents, cryosurgery, laser excision or surgical excision.

Vesiculobullous disorders, such as erythema multiforme, pemphigoid and pemphigus, may present as red lesions (Article 2), especially localized oral purpura, which presents with blood blisters (Figure 12). Specialist referral is usually indicated.

Reactive lesions

Reactive lesions that can be red are usually persistent soft lumps (Figures 13 and 14) which include:
■ Pyogenic granulomas; and
■ Peripheral giant cell granulomas.

Specialist referral is usually indicated.

Atrophic lesions

The most important red lesion is erythroplasia, since it is often dysplastic (see below). Geographic tongue also causes red lesions (see above). Desquamative gingivitis is a frequent cause of red gingivae (Figure 15), which is almost invariably caused by lichen planus or pemphigoid, and iron or vitamin deficiency states may cause glossitis (Figure 16) or other red lesions.

Erythroplakia (erythroplasia)

Erythroplasia is a rare condition defined as 'any lesion of the oral mucosa that presents as bright red velvety plaques which cannot be characterized clinically or pathologically as any other recognizable condition'.

Mainly seen in elderly males, it is far less common than leukoplakia, but far more likely to be dysplastic or undergo malignant transformation.

Clinical features

Erythroplakia is seen most commonly on the soft palate, floor of mouth or buccal mucosa. Some erythroplakias are associated with white patches, and are then termed speckled leukoplakia (Figure 17).

Diagnosis

Biopsy to assess the degree of epithelial dysplasia and

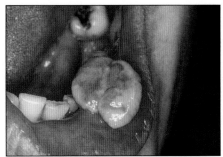
Figure 13. Pyogenic granuloma, lower lip.

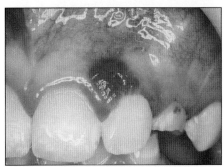
Figure 14. Pyogenic epulis.

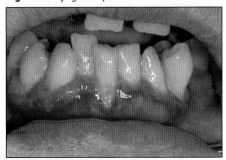
Figure 15. Desquamative gingivitis.

exclude a diagnosis of carcinoma.

Prognosis

Erythroplasia has areas of dysplasia, carcinoma *in situ*, or invasive carcinoma in most cases. Carcinomas are seen 17 times more often in erythroplakia than in leukoplakia and these are therefore the most potentially malignant of all oral mucosal lesions.

Management

Erythroplastic lesions are usually (at least 85%) severely dysplastic or frankly malignant. Any causal factor, such as tobacco use, should be stopped, and lesions removed.

There is no hard evidence as to the ideal frequency of follow-up, but it has been suggested that patients with mucosal potentially malignant lesions be re-examined:
- Within 1 month;
- At 3 months;
- At 6 months;
- At 12 months and
- Annually thereafter.

Purpura (bleeding into the skin and mucosa) is usually caused by:
- Trauma, occasional small petechiae are seen at the occlusal line in perfectly healthy people;
- Localized oral purpura or angina bullosa haemorrhagica is an idiopathic, fairly common cause of blood blisters, often in the soft palate, in older people (Figure 12). Sometimes the use of a corticosteroid inhaler precipitates this;
- Thrombocytopenia can result in red or brown pinpoint lesions (petechiae) or diffuse bruising (ecchymoses) at sites of trauma, such as the palate;
- Suction (eg fellatio may produce bruising in the soft palate).

Diagnosis

Diagnosis of red lesions is mainly clinical but lesions should also be sought elsewhere, especially on the skin or other mucosae.

It may be necessary to take a blood picture (including full blood count and platelet count), and assess haemostatic function or exclude haematinic deficiencies. Investigations needed may include other haematological tests and/or biopsy or imaging.

Management

Treatment is usually of the underlying cause, or surgery.

Hyperpigmentation

Oral mucosal discoloration may be superficial (extrinsic) or due to deep (intrinsic – in or beneath mucosa) causes and ranges from brown to black.

Causes of **extrinsic discoloration** include:
- Habits such as tobacco or betel use;
- Coloured foods or drinks (such as liquorice, beetroot, red wine, coffee and tea);
- Drugs (such as chlorhexidine, iron salts, crack cocaine, minocycline, bismuth subsalicylate and lansoprazole).

Black hairy tongue (Figure 18) is one extrinsic type of discoloration seen especially in patients on a soft diet,

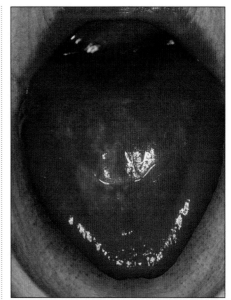
Figure 16. Atrophic glossitis.

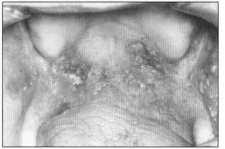
Figure 17. Erythroplasia in soft palate complex.

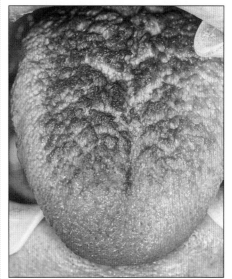
Figure 18. Black hairy tongue.

smokers, and those with dry mouth or poor oral hygiene. The best that can usually be done is to avoid the cause where known, and to advise the patient to brush the tongue or use a tongue-scraper.

Causes of **Intrinsic discoloration** are summarized in Table 3.

Localized areas of pigmentation may be caused mainly by:
■ *Amalgam tattoo* (embedded amalgam). Typically, this is a single blue-black macule in the mandibular gingivae, or at least close to the scar of an apicectomy (Figures 19 and 20), or where amalgam has accidentally been introduced into a wound, is painless, and does not change in size or colour. A lesion suspected to be an amalgam tattoo is best radiographed first to see if there is radio-opaque material present, though not all are radio-opaque. If the lesion is *not* radio-opaque, it is best biopsied to exclude naevi or melanoma. Similar lesions can be caused by other foreign bodies (eg graphite tattoo), local irritation or inflammation.
■ *Melanotic macules* are usually flat, single brown collections of melanin-containing cells, seen particularly on the vermilion border of the lip (Figure 21) and on the palate. If there is any doubt over the diagnosis they are best removed to exclude melanoma.
■ *Naevi* are blue-black, often papular, lesions formed from increased melanin-containing cells (naevus cells) seen particularly on the palate. They are best removed to exclude melanoma.
■ *Pigmentary incontinence* may be seen in some inflammatory lesions, such as lichen planus, especially in smokers.
■ *Malignant melanoma* is rare, seen usually in the palate (Figure 22) or maxillary gingivae. Features suggestive of malignancy include a rapid increase in size, change in colour, ulceration, pain, the occurrence of satellite pigmented spots or regional lymph node enlargement. Incisional biopsy to confirm the diagnosis followed by radical excision is indicated.
■ *Kaposi's sarcoma* is usually a purple lesion seen mainly in the palate (Figure 23) or gingivae of HIV-infected and other immunocompromised people.

Keypoints: single hyperpigmented lesions
■ If the lesion could be an amalgam tattoo, consider taking a radiograph;
■ If the lesion is radio-opaque, it is probably an amalgam tattoo and should be left alone;
■ If the lesion is not radio-opaque, or if it was not initially considered likely to be an amalgam tattoo, biopsy it.

Generalized pigmentation, often mainly affecting the gingivae (Figure 24) is common in people of colour, and is racial and due to melanin. Seen mainly in black and ethnic minority groups, it can also be noted in some fairly light-skinned people. Such pigmentation may be first noted by

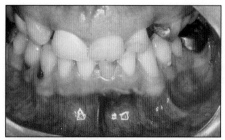
Figure 19. Amalgam tattoo.

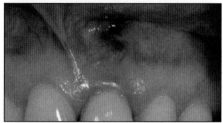
Figure 20. Amalgam tattoo.

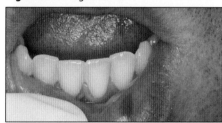
Figure 21. Melantonic macule, lower labial mucosa.

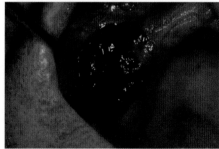
Figure 22. Malignant melanoma, palate.

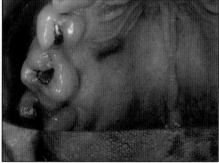
Figure 23. Kaposi's sarcoma, palate.

the patient in adult life and then incorrectly assumed to be acquired.

In all other patients with widespread intrinsic pigmentation, systemic causes should be excluded. These may include:
- Drugs
  - Tobacco, which can also cause intrinsic hyperpigmentation – smoker's melanosis (Figure 25);
  - Antimalarials, oral contraceptive pill, anticonvulsants, minocycline, phenothiazines, gold, busulphan and other drugs;
  - Heavy metals (such as mercury, lead and bismuth) not used therapeutically now, rarely cause pigmentation through industrial exposure;
- Pregnancy;
- Hypoadrenalism (Addison's disease). Hyperpigmentation in this is generalized but most obvious in normally pigmented areas (eg the nipples, genitalia), skin flexures, and sites of trauma. The mouth may show patchy hyperpigmentation. Patients also typically have weakness, weight loss, and hypotension.

Diagnosis

The nature of oral hyperpigmentation can sometimes only be established after further investigation.

In patients with localized hyperpigmentation, in order to exclude melanoma, radiographs may be helpful (they can sometimes show a foreign body) and biopsy may be indicated, particularly where there is a solitary raised lesion, a rapid increase in size, change in colour, ulceration, pain, evidence of satellite pigmented spots or regional lymph node enlargement. If early detection of oral melanomas is to be achieved, all pigmented oral cavity lesions should be viewed with suspicion. The consensus of opinion is that a lesion with clinical features, as above, seriously suggestive of malignant melanoma, are best biopsied at the time of definitive operation.

In patients with generalized or multiple hyperpigmentation, Specialist referral is indicated.

Management

Management is of the underlying condition.

Patients to refer:
- Erythroplasia/erythroplakia – in view of high risk of malignant transformation;
- Squamous carcinoma;

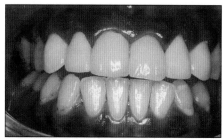

Figure 24. Racial pigmentation.

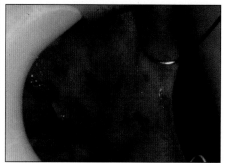

Figure 25. Smoking-induced melanosis.

Localized
- Amalgam or other tattoo
- Naevus
- Melanotic macule
- Neoplasms (eg Malignant melanoma or Kaposi's sarcoma)
- Pigmentary incontinence
- Peutz-Jegher's syndrome

Generalized
- Racial pigmentation
- Localized irritation, eg tobacco or betel
- Drugs, eg antimalarials
- Pregnancy/oral contraceptive pill
- Addison's disease (hypoadrenalism)

Table 3. Main causes of intrinsic mucosal hyperpigmentation.

- Melanoma;
- Kaposi's sarcoma;
- Wegener granulomatosis in view of associated systemic disease.

Orofacial Sensation and Movement

8

Disorders of orofacial sensation and movement

Sensory innervation of the mouth, face and most of the scalp depends on the fifth cranial (trigeminal) nerve, so that disease affecting this nerve can cause sensory loss or orofacial pain, or indeed both, sometimes with serious implications. The trigeminal nerve also provides motor supply to the muscles of mastication.

The facial (seventh cranial) nerve controls the muscles of facial expression, so that lesions of the nerve (lower motor neurone lesions) or its central connections (upper motor neurone lesions) can lead to facial weakness. The facial nerve also carries nerve impulses to the tear glands, to the salivary glands, and to the stapedius muscle of the stirrup bone (the stapes) in the middle ear and also transmits taste from the anterior tongue, so that lesions involving this nerve may also affect taste and hearing, lacrimation and salivation.

It is evident, therefore, that dental surgeons should be able to carry out examination of these and other cranial nerves as shown in Table 1.

The olfactory nerve (cranial nerve I)

Bilateral anosmia is common after head injuries involving the anterior cranial fossa, but in practice the patient may complain of loss of taste rather than sense of smell.

An olfactory lesion is confirmed by inability to smell substances such as orange or peppermint oil. Ammoniacal solutions or other substances with a pungent odour must not be used since they stimulate the trigeminal rather than the olfactory nerve thereby giving a false positive result.

The optic nerve (cranial nerve II)

Blindness or defects of visual fields are caused by ocular, optic nerve or cortical damage but the type of defect varies according to the site and extent of the lesion.

If there is a complete lesion of one optic nerve that eye is totally blind, there is no direct reaction of the pupil to light (loss of constriction) and, if a light is shone into the affected eye, the pupil of the *unaffected* eye also fails to respond (loss of the consensual reflex). However, the nerves to the affected eye that are responsible for pupil constriction run in the IIIrd cranial nerve and should be intact. If, therefore, a light is shone into the unaffected eye, the pupil of the affected eye also constricts, even though it is sightless.

Lesions of the optic tract, chiasma, radiation or optic cortex cause various defects involving both visual fields but without total field loss on either side.

An ophthalmological opinion should always be obtained if there is any suggestion of a visual field defect.

The oculomotor nerve (cranial nerve III)

The oculomotor nerve supplies the muscle that raises the upper eyelid, most of the orbital muscles that move the eye (except the lateral rectus and superior oblique), and the ciliary muscle and pupil constrictor.

Normally, the medial rectus (supplied by the IIIrd nerve) moves the eye medially (adducts). The lateral rectus (VIth nerve) abducts the eye. When the eye is abducted it is elevated by the superior rectus (IIIrd nerve) and depressed by the inferior rectus (IIIrd nerve). The adducted eye is depressed by the superior oblique muscle (IVth nerve) and elevated by the inferior oblique (IIIrd nerve).

Disruption of the oculomotor nerve therefore causes:
- Ptosis (drooping upper eyelid);
- Double vision and divergent squint. The affected eye points downwards and laterally - 'down and out' in all directions except when looking towards the affected side;
- Paralysis of internal, upward and downward rotation of the eye;
- A dilated pupil which fails to constrict on accommodation or when light is shone either on to the affected eye (negative direct light reaction) or into the unaffected eye (negative consensual light reaction).

The trochlear nerve (cranial nerve IV)

The trochlear nerve supplies only the superior oblique muscle which moves the eye downwards and medially towards the nose.

	Nerve	Examination	Examination findings in lesions
I	Olfactory	Sense of smell	Impaired sense of smell for common odours (stimuli used should be non-irritant and readily identifiable eg oil of cloves; do not use ammonia).
II	Optic	Visual acuity Visual fields Pupil responses	Visual acuity reduced using Snellen types ± ophthalmoscopy: nystagmus. Visual fields by confrontation impaired; may be impaired pupil responses.
III	Oculomotor	Eye movements Pupil responses	Diplopia; strabismus; eye looks down and laterally; movements impaired; ptosis; pupil dilated. Pupil reactions: direct reflex impaired but consensual reflex intact.
IV	Trochlear	Eye movements Pupil responses?	Diplopia, particularly on looking down; strabismus; no ptosis; pupil normal and normal reactivity.
V	Trigeminal	Sensation over face Corneal reflex Jaw jerk Taste sensation	Reduced sensation over face; ± corneal reflex impaired; ± taste sensation impaired; motor power of masticatory muscles reduced, with weakness on opening jaw; jaw jerk impaired; muscle wasting.
VI	Abducens	Eye movements Pupil responses?	Diplopia; strabismus; eye movements impaired to affected side; pupil normal and normal reactivity.
VII	Facial	Motor power of facial muscles Corneal reflex Taste sensation	Impaired motor power of facial muscles on smiling, blowing out cheeks, showing teeth, etc; corneal reflex reduced; ± taste sensation impaired.
VIII	Vestibulo-cochlear	Whisper in ear and ask patient to repeat Remember to cover the other ear	Impaired hearing; impaired balance; ± nystagmus.
IX	Glosso-pharyngeal	Gag reflex Taste sensation Voice	Reduced gag reflex; deviation of uvula; reduced taste sensation; voice may have nasal tone.
X	Vagal	Gag reflex Voice	Reduced gag reflex; deviation of palate; voice hoarse.
XI	Accessory	Ability to shrug shoulders and rotate head against resistance	Motor power of trapezius and sternomastoid reduced.
XII	Hypoglossal	Tongue protrusion	Motor power of tongue impaired, with abnormal speech; ± fasciculation, wasting, ipsilateral deviation on protrusion

Table 1. Examination of cranial nerves.

The lesion is characterized by:
- The head tilted away from the affected side;
- Diplopia, maximal on looking downwards and inwards;
- Normal pupils.

There is often damage to the IIIrd and VIth nerves as well.

Damage to the trochlear nerve causes serious disability, because there is diplopia maximal on looking down and the patient may therefore have difficulty reading, going down stairs or seeing obstructions on the ground.

The trigeminal nerve (cranial nerve V)

The trigeminal nerve supplies sensation over the whole face apart from the angle of the jaw, and the front of the scalp back to a line drawn across the vertex, between the ears. It also supplies sensation to most of the mucosa of the oral cavity, conjunctivae, nose, tympanic membrane and sinuses.

The motor division of the trigeminal nerve supplies the muscles of mastication (masseter, medial and lateral pterygoids, temporalis, mylohyoid and anterior belly of the digastric).

Taste fibres from the anterior two-thirds of the tongue, and secretomotor fibres to the submandibular and sublingual salivary glands and lacrimal glands, are also carried in branches of the trigeminal nerve.

Damage to a sensory branch of the trigeminal nerve causes hypoaesthesia in its area of distribution; infection, such as with herpes zoster (Figure 1), causes pain. Lesions of the sensory part of the trigeminal nerve initially result in a diminishing response to pin-prick to the skin and, later, complete anaesthesia. Lesions involving the ophthalmic division also cause corneal anaesthesia: this is tested by *gently* touching the cornea with a wisp of cotton wool twisted to a point. Normally this procedure causes a blink, but not if the cornea is anaesthetic and the patient does not see the cotton wool.

It is important, with patients complaining of facial anaesthesia, to test all areas, but particularly the corneal reflex with a wisp of cotton wool, and the reaction to pin-prick over the angle of the mandible. If the patient complains of complete facial or hemifacial anaesthesia, but the corneal reflex is retained or there is anaesthesia over the angle of the mandible, then the symptoms are probably functional rather than organic as the skin overlying the angle of the mandible is not supplied by the trigeminal nerve.

Taste can be tested with sweet, salt, sour or bitter substances (sugar, salt, lemon juice or vinegar) carefully applied to the dorsum of the tongue, or by asking the patient to touch his tongue between the terminals of a pocket torch battery: this normally gives a tingling sensation and a characteristic metallic taste.

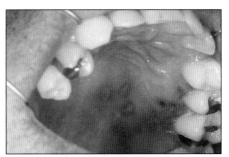

Figure 1. Herpes zoster, palate.

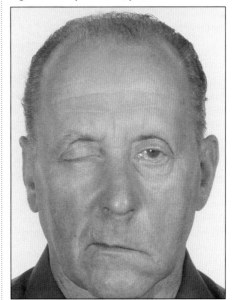

Figure 2. Facial nerve palsy.

Damage to the motor part of the trigeminal nerve can be difficult to detect and is usually asymptomatic if unilateral, but the jaw may deviate towards the affected side on opening. It is easier to detect motor weakness by asking the patient to open the jaw against resistance, rather than by trying to test the strength of closure.

The abducens nerve (cranial nerve VI)

The abducens nerve supplies only one eye muscle, the lateral rectus. Lesions comprise:
- Deviation of the affected eye towards the nose;
- Paralysis of abduction of the eye;
- Convergent squint with diplopia maximal on looking laterally towards the affected side;
- Normal pupils.

Lesions of the abducens can, however, be surprisingly disabling.

The facial nerve (cranial nerve VII)

The facial nerve carries:
■ The motor supply to the muscles of facial expression;
■ Taste sensation from the anterior two-thirds of the tongue (via the chorda tympani);
■ Secretomotor fibres to the submandibular and sublingual salivary glands;
■ Secretomotor fibres to the lacrimal glands;
■ Branches to the stapedius muscle in the middle ear.

The neurones supplying the lower part of the face receive upper motor neurones (UMNs) from the contralateral motor cortex, whereas the neurones to the upper face receive bilateral UMN innervation.

An UMN lesion therefore causes unilateral facial palsy with some sparing of the frontalis and orbicularis oculi muscles because of the bilateral cortical representation. Furthermore, although voluntary facial movements are impaired, the face may still move with emotional responses, for example on laughing. Paresis of the ipsilateral arm (monoparesis) or arm and leg (hemiparesis), or dysphasia may be associated because of more extensive cerebrocortical damage.

Lower motor neurone (LMN)facial palsy is characterized by unilateral paralysis of all muscles of facial expression (Figure 2) for both voluntary and emotional responses. The forehead is unfurrowed and the patient unable to close the eye on that side. Attempted closure causes the eye to roll upwards (Bell's sign). Tears tend to overflow on to the cheek (epiphora), the corner of the mouth droops and the nasolabial fold is obliterated. Saliva may dribble from the commissure and may cause angular stomatitis. Food collects in the vestibule and plaque accumulates on the teeth on the affected side. Depending on the site of the lesion, other defects, such as loss of taste or hyperacusis, may be associated.

In facial palsy, facial weakness is demonstrated by asking the patient to:
■ Close the eyes against resistance;
■ Raise the eyebrows;
■ Raise the lips to show the teeth;
■ Try to whistle.

The following investigations may be indicated:
■ Full neurological examination, looking particularly for signs suggesting a central lesion, such as:
  – hemiparesis;

Extracranial
Trauma (eg surgical; fractures) to inferior dental, lingual, mental or infraorbital nerves
Inflammatory
  – osteomyelitis
Neoplastic carcinoma of antrum or nasopharynx
  – metastatic tumours
  – leukaemic deposits

Intracranial
Trauma (eg surgical; fractures) – eg surgical treatment of trigeminal neuralgia
Inflammatory
  – multiple sclerosis, neurosyphilis, HIV infection
  – sarcoidosis
Neoplastic cerebral tumours
Syringobulbia
Vascular
  – cerebrovascular disease
  – aneurysms
Bone disease
  – Paget's disease
Drugs
  – Labetalol

Benign trigeminal neuropathy
Idiopathic
Psychogenic
Hysteria
  – Hyperventilation syndrome

Organic disease

Table 2. Causes of sensory loss in the trigeminal area.

  – tremor;
  – loss of balance;
  – involvement of the Vth, VIth or VIIIth cranial nerves.
■ Imaging with MRI, or CT, of the internal auditory meatus, cerebellopontine angle and mastoid may be needed to exclude an organic lesion such as a tumour, particularly in progressive facial palsy.
■ Study of evoked potentials to assess the degree of nerve damage. Facial nerve stimulation or needle electromyography may be useful, as may electrogustometry, nerve excitability tests, electromyography and electroneuronography;

- Blood pressure measurement (to exclude hypertension);
- Blood tests that may include:
  - fasting blood sugar levels (to exclude diabetes);
  - tests for HSV or other virus infections such as HIV may need to be considered;
  - serum angiotensin converting enzyme levels as a screen for sarcoidosis;
  - serum antinuclear antibodies to exclude connective tissue disease;
  - in some areas, Lyme disease (tick-borne infection with *Borrelia burgdorferi*) should be excluded by ELISA test;
- Schirmer's test for lacrimation, carried out by gently placing a strip of filter paper on the lower conjunctival sac and comparing the wetting of the paper with that on the other side;
- Test for loss of hearing;
- Test for taste loss by applying sugar, salt, lemon juice or vinegar on the tongue and asking the patient to identify each of them;
- Aural examination for discharge and other signs of middle ear disease;
- Lumbar puncture occasionally.

The vestibulocochlear nerve (cranial nerve VIII)

The vestibulocochlear nerve has two components:
- The vestibular (concerned with appreciation of the movements and position of the head); and
- The cochlear (hearing).

Lesions of this nerve may cause loss of hearing, vertigo or ringing in the ears (tinnitus).

An ENT opinion should be obtained if a lesion of the vestibulocochlear nerve is suspected, as special tests are needed for diagnosis.

The glossopharyngeal nerve (cranial nerve IX)

The glossopharyngeal nerve carries:
- The sensory supply to the posterior third of the tongue and pharynx;
- Taste sensation from the posterior third of the tongue;
- Motor supply to the stylopharyngeus;
- Secretomotor fibres to the parotid.

Symptoms resulting from a IXth nerve lesion include impaired pharyngeal sensation so that the gag reflex may be weakened; the two sides should always be compared. Lesions of the glossopharyngeal are usually associated with lesions of the vagus, accessory and hypoglossal nerves (bulbar palsy).

Upper motor neurone lesion:
- Cerebrovascular event
- Trauma
- Tumour
- Infection
- Multiple sclerosis

Lower motor neurone lesion:
Systemic infection
- Bell's palsy (herpes simplex virus usually)
- Varicella-Zoster virus infection (+/- Ramsay-Hunt syndrome)
- Lyme disease (*B. burgdorferii*)
- HIV infection

Middle ear disease
- Otitis media
- Cholesteatoma

Lesion of skull base
- Fracture
- Infection

Parotid lesion
- Tumour

Trauma to branch of facial nerve

Table 3. Causes of facial palsy. (Reproduced from Scully C. *Medical Problems in Dentistry*. Elsevier, 2010.

The vagus nerve (cranial nerve X)

The vagus has a wide parasympathetic distribution to the viscera of the thorax and upper abdomen but is also the motor supply to some soft palate, pharyngeal and laryngeal muscles.

Lesions of the vagus are rare in isolation but have the following effects:
- Impaired gag reflex;
- The soft palate moves towards the unaffected side when the patient is asked to say 'aah';
- Hoarse voice;
- Bovine cough.

The accessory nerve (cranial nerve XI)

The accessory nerve is the motor supply to the sternomastoid and trapezius muscles. Lesions are often associated with damage to the IXth and Xth nerves and cause:
- Weakness of the sternomastoid (weakness on turning the head away from the affected side); and
- Weakness of the trapezius on shrugging the shoulders.

Testing this nerve is useful in differentiating patients with genuine palsies from those with functional complaints. In an accessory nerve lesion there is weakness on turning the head away from the affected side. Those shamming paralysis often simulate weakness when turning the head towards the 'affected' side.

The hypoglossal nerve (cranial nerve XII)

The hypoglossal nerve is the motor supply to the muscles of the tongue. Lesions cause:
■ Dysarthria (difficulty in speaking) – particularly for lingual sounds; and
■ Deviation of the tongue towards the affected side, on protrusion.

The hypoglossal nerve may be affected in its intra- or extracranial course. Intracranial lesions typically cause bulbar palsy. In an upper motor neurone lesion the tongue is spastic but not wasted; in a lower motor neurone lesion there is wasting and fibrillation of the affected side of the tongue.

Facial sensory loss

Normal facial sensation is important to protect the skin, oral mucosa and especially cornea from damage. Lesions affecting the sensory part of the trigeminal nerve initially result in a diminishing response to light touch (cotton wool) and pin-prick (gently pricking the skin with a sterile pin or needle without drawing blood) and, later, there is complete anaesthesia. Facial sensory awareness may be:
■ Completely lost (**anaesthesia**); or
■ Partially lost (**hypoaesthesia**).

The term **paraesthesia** does not mean loss of sensation, rather it means abnormal sensation.

Lesions of a sensory branch of the trigeminal nerve may cause anaesthesia in the distribution of the affected branch. Facial sensory loss may be caused by intracranial or, more frequently, by extracranial lesions of the trigeminal nerve and may lead to corneal, facial or oral ulceration (Table 2).

If the patient complains of complete facial or hemifacial anaesthesia, but the corneal reflex is retained, then the symptoms are probably functional (non-organic) or due to benign trigeminal neuropathy. If the patient complains of complete facial or hemifacial anaesthesia and there is apparent anaesthesia over the angle of the mandible (an area not innervated by the trigeminal nerve), then the symptoms are almost certainly functional (non-organic).

Extracranial causes of facial sensory loss are shown in Table 2. The mandibular division or its branches may be traumatized by inferior alveolar local analgesic injections, fractures or surgery (particularly surgical extraction of lower third

	UMN lesions	LMN lesions
Emotional movements of face	Retained	Lost
Blink reflex	Retained	Lost
Ability to wrinkle forehead	Retained	Lost
Drooling from commissure	Uncommon	Common
Lacrimation, taste or hearing	Unaffected	May be affected

Table 4. Differentiation of upper (UMN) from lower motor neurone (LMN) lesions of the facial nerve.

molars or osteotomies). Occasionally, there is dehiscence of the mental foramen in an atrophic mandible leading to anaesthesia of the lower lip on the affected side, as a result of pressure from the denture. The inferior alveolar or lingual nerves may be damaged, especially during removal of lower third molars, particularly when the lingual split technique is used. Osteomyelitis or tumour deposits in the mandible may affect the inferior alveolar nerve to cause labial anaesthesia.

Nasopharyngeal carcinomas may invade the pharyngeal wall to infiltrate the mandibular division of the trigeminal nerve, causing pain and sensory loss and, by occluding the Eustachian tube, deafness (Trotter syndrome).

Damage to branches of the maxillary division of the trigeminal may be caused by trauma (middle-third facial fractures) or a tumour such as carcinoma of the maxillary antrum.

Intracranial causes of facial sensory loss

Intracranial causes of sensory loss are uncommon but serious and include:
■ Multiple sclerosis;
■ Brain tumours;
■ Syringobulbia;
■ Sarcoidosis;
■ Infections (eg HIV).

Since other cranial nerves are anatomically close, there may be associated neurological deficits. In posterior fossa lesions, for example, there may be cerebellar features such as ataxia. In middle cranial fossa lesions, there may be associated neurological deficits affecting cranial nerve VI (abducens nerve), resulting in impaired lateral movement of the eye.

Benign trigeminal neuropathy

This is a transient sensory loss in one or more divisions of

Muscles	Lacrimation paralysed	Hyperacusis	Sense of taste	Other features	Probable site of lesion	Type of lesion
Lower face	N	–	N	Emotional movement retained + monoparesis or hemiparesis + aphasia	Upper motor neurone (UMN)	Stroke (cerebrovascular event) Brain tumour Trauma HIV infection
All facial muscles	↓	+	↓	+ VIth nerve damage	Lower motor neurone (LMN) Facial nucleus	Multiple sclerosis
All facial muscles	↓	+	↓	+ VIIIth nerve damage	Between nucleus and geniculate ganglion	Fractured base of skull Posterior cranial fossa tumours Sarcoidosis
All facial muscles	N	+	N or ↓	–	Between geniculate ganglion and stylomastoid canal	Otitis media Cholesteatoma Mastoiditis
All facial muscles	N	–	N	–	In tylomastoid canal or extracranially	Bell's palsy Trauma Local analgesia (eg misplaced inferior dental block) Parotid malignant neoplasm Guillain-Barre syndrome
Isolated facial muscles	N	–	N	–	Branch of facial nerve extracranially	Trauma Local analgesia

Table 5. Localization of site of lesion in and causes of unilateral facial palsy. N = normal; + = present; ↓ = reduced.

the trigeminal nerve which seldom occurs until the second decade. The corneal reflex is not affected. The aetiology is unknown, though some patients prove to have connective tissue disorder.

Psychogenic causes of facial sensory loss

Hysteria, and particularly hyperventilation syndrome, may underlie some causes of facial anaesthesia.

Organic causes of facial sensory loss

Include diabetes or connective tissue disorders.

Diagnosis in facial sensory loss

In view of the potential seriousness of facial sensory loss, care should be taken to exclude local causes and a full neurological assessment must be undertaken. Since, in the case of posterior or middle cranial fossa lesions, other cranial nerves are anatomically close, there may be associated neurological deficits. Thus, in the absence of any obvious local cause, or if there are additional neurological deficits, patients should be referred for a specialist opinion.

Management of patients with facial sensory loss

If the cornea is anaesthetic, a protective eye pad should be worn and a tarsorrhaphy (an operation to unite the upper and lower eyelids) may be indicated since the protective corneal reflex is lost and the cornea may be traumatized.

Orofacial movement disorders

The facial nerve not only carries nerve impulses to the muscles of the face, but also to the tear glands, to the salivary glands, and to the stapedius muscle of the stirrup bone (the stapes) in the middle ear. It also transmits taste from the anterior tongue. Since the function of the facial nerve is so complex, many symptoms may occur if it is disrupted.

The main movement disorder is facial palsy, which can have a range of causes (Table 3) and may be due to UMN or LMN lesions, as discussed above.

The common cause of facial palsy is stroke, an UMN, and this is a medical emergency for which specialist care is indicated. The GDP should be able to differentiate UMN from LMN lesions (see above and Table 4).

The facial nerve should be tested, by examining facial movements, and other functions mediated by the nerve. Movement of the mouth as patients speak is important, especially when they allow themselves the luxury of some emotional expression. The upper part of the face is bilaterally innervated and thus loss of wrinkles on one half of the forehead, or absence of blinking, suggest a lesion is in the lower motor neurone.

If the patient is asked to close his/her eyes, any palsy may become obvious, with the affected eyelids failing to close and the globe turning up so that only the white of the eye is showing (Bell's sign). Weakness of orbicularis muscles with sufficient strength to close the eyes can be compared with the normal side by asking the patient to close his/her eyes tight and observing the degree of force required to part the eyelids. If the patient is asked to wrinkle his/her forehead, weakness can be detected by the difference between the two sides.

Lower face

Round the mouth movements are best examined by asking the patient to:
- Smile;
- Bare the teeth;
- Purse the lips; or
- Blow out the cheeks.

Corneal reflex

This depends on the integrity of the trigeminal and facial nerve, either of which being defective will give a negative response. It is important to test facial light touch sensation in all areas, but particularly the corneal reflex. Lesions involving the ophthalmic division cause corneal anaesthesia, which is tested by gently touching the cornea with a wisp of cotton wool twisted to a point. Normally, this procedure causes a blink but, if the cornea is anaesthetic (or if there is facial palsy), no blink follows, provided that the patient does not actually see the cotton wool.

Taste

Unilateral loss of taste associated with facial palsy indicates that the facial nerve is damaged proximal to the chorda tympani.

Hearing

Hyperacusis may be caused by paralysis of the stapedius muscle and this suggests the lesion is proximal to the nerve to stapedius.

Lacrimation

This is tested by hooking a Schirmer strip in the lower conjunctival fornix. The strip should dampen to at least 15 mm in five minutes if tear production is normal. The contralateral eye serves as a control (Schirmer test). Secretion is diminished in proximal lesions of the facial nerve, such as those involving the geniculate ganglion or in the internal auditory meatus.

Bell's palsy

Bell's palsy is the most common *acute* LMN paralysis (palsy) of the face. There is inflammation of the facial nerve which may be immunologically mediated and associated with infection, commonly herpes simplex virus (HSV), leading to demyelination and oedema, usually in the stylomastoid canal.

The condition is usually seen in young adults; predisposing factors, found in a minority of cases, include:
- Pregnancy;
- Hypertension;
- Diabetes; or
- Lymphoma.

Aetiopathogenesis

LMN facial palsy is usually associated with infections:
- Mainly with herpes simplex virus (HSV);
- Rarely, another virus such as:
  - Varicella-Zoster virus (VZV) infection;
  - Epstein-Barr virus (EBV) infection;
  - Cytomegalovirus (CMV) infection;

– Human herpesvirus-6 infection;
– HIV infection.
■ Occasionally with bacterial infections such as:
– Otitis media;
– Lyme disease.

Clinical features

Damage to the facial nerve may result in twitching, weakness, or paralysis of the face, in dryness of the eye or the mouth, or in disturbance of taste.

There is:
■ Acute onset of paralysis over a few hours, maximal within 48 hours;
■ Paralysis of upper and lower face, usually only unilaterally;
■ Diminished blinking and the absence of tearing. These together result in corneal drying, erosion and ulceration and the possible loss of the eye;
■ Occasionally:
– Pain around the ear or jaw may precede the palsy by a day or two;
– There may be apparent facial numbness, but sensation is actually intact on testing;
– If the lesion is located proximal to the stylomastoid canal, there may *also* be (Table 5):
– Hyperacusis (raised hearing sensitivity; loss of function of nerve to stapedius); or
– Loss of taste (loss of function of the chorda tympani); or
– Loss of lacrimation. Up to 10% of patients have a positive family history and a similar percentage suffer recurrent episodes.

Diagnosis of Bell's palsy

The *history* should be directed to exclude facial palsy caused by other factors, such as:
■ Stroke;
■ Trauma to the facial nerve (eg in parotid region or to the base of skull or underwater diving (barotraumas);
■ Tumours close to facial nerve (eg acoustic neuroma;
■ Facial nerve inflammatory disorders:
– Multiple sclerosis;
– Connective tissue disease;
– Sarcoidosis;
– Melkersson-Rosenthal syndrome;
– Viral infections (HSV, VZV, EBV, CMV, HIV);
– Bacterial infections;
– Middle ear infections (eg otitis media);
– Lyme disease (from camping or walking in areas that contain deer ticks that transmit *Borrelia burgdorferii*

The *examination* and investigations are discussed above.

Management of Bell's palsy

Treatment with systemic corticosteroids results in 80–90% complete recovery. There is thus a strong argument for treating all patients with prednisolone 20 mg four times a day for 5 days, then tailing off over the succeeding 4 days.

Since HSV is frequently implicated, antivirals may be used. However, despite the fact that HSV is frequently implicated, there is no evidence of a benefit of adding aciclovir.

Key points: Bell's palsy

■ This is fairly common;
■ It affects only the facial nerve;
■ It may be caused by herpes simplex virus, or other infections;
■ It is not contagious;
■ It disproportionately attacks pregnant women and people who have diabetes, influenza, a cold, or immune problems;
■ There are usually no serious long-term consequences;
■ Corticosteroids and antivirals are used;
■ Most patients begin to get significantly better within 2 weeks, and about 80% recover completely within 3 months;
■ It rarely recurs, but can in 5–10% of cases.

Key points for patients: Bell's palsy

■ This is fairly common;
■ It affects only the facial nerve; there are no brain or other neurological problems;
■ It may be caused by herpes simplex virus, or other infections;
■ It is not contagious;
■ There are usually no serious long-term consequences;
■ X-rays and blood tests *may* be required;
■ Treatment takes time and patience; corticosteroids and antivirals are used;
■ Most patients recover completely within 3 months;
■ It rarely recurs.

Websites and patient information

http://www.entnet.org
http://www.ninds.nih.gov/health_and_medical/
disorders/bells_doc.htm
http://www.bellspalsy.ws/

Patients to refer:

Any patient with a cranial nerve defect requiring further investigation is outwith the scope of primary dental care.

Orofacial Pain

9

Pain

Pain in the teeth, mouth, face or head usually has a *local* cause – often the sequelae of dental caries (odontogenic pain) – but *psychogenic, neurological, vascular* and conditions where pain is referred from elsewhere may be responsible (Table 1).

Dental staff will be well versed in pain of local cause and therefore this article discusses mainly the conditions in which specialist help may be indicated. Many of the conditions discussed in previous articles in this series may cause pain.

The real significance to the patient of orofacial pain, apart from the pain itself, can range from the benign to potentially lethal conditions. Some orofacial pain or headaches have an obvious but relatively unimportant cause (eg a hangover – caused mainly by the acetaldehyde resulting from metabolism of alcohol); other types of pain have no obvious underlying organic pathology (and are thus termed medically unexplained symptoms (MUS), eg atypical facial pain); some can threaten important faculties such as sight (eg giant cell arteritis), or even life (eg brain tumours).

Diagnosis of orofacial pain

The history is the most important means of diagnosing orofacial pain (Figure 1).

In order to differentiate the widely disparate causes, it is essential to determine keypoints about the pain, especially:
- **Location:** Valuable information can be obtained by asking if the pain is localized or diffuse, and watching the patient's reaction. For example, patients frequently point with one finger when describing pain of dental causes or trigeminal neuralgia, but atypical facial pain is much more diffuse, and may radiate across the midline.
- **Character:** Patients should be asked about the severity and character of the pain, ie whether the pain is 'sharp', 'dull', 'aching', 'throbbing' or 'shooting'. However, bear in mind that patients often have difficulty finding adequate descriptors, and therefore it may be necessary to ask leading questions. Ask the patient to rate the pain severity on a scale of zero (no pain) to 10 (most severe pain that

Local disorders
Teeth and supporting tissues:
    Jaws;
    Maxillary antrum;
    Salivary glands;
    Pharynx;
    Eyes.
Possible psychogenic causes
    Chronic idiopathic facial pain (atypical facial pain);
    Burning mouth syndrome;
    Temporomandibular pain-dysfunction.
Neurological disorders
    Idiopathic trigeminal neuralgia;
    Malignant neoplasms involving the trigeminal nerve;
    Glossopharyngeal neuralgia;
    Herpes zoster (including post-herpetic neuralgia);
    Multiple sclerosis.
Vascular disorders
    Migraine;
    Periodic migrainous neuralgia;
    Giant cell arteritis.
Referred pain
    Nasopharyngeal;
    Ocular;
    Aural;
    Cardiorespiratory:
    – Angina;
    – Lesions in the neck or chest (including lung cancer).

Table 1. Causes of orofacial pain.

the patient has experienced), or ask them to mark this on a line divided into 10 equal sections (visual analogue scale) or use an assessment instrument such as the McGill Pain Questionnaire. These 'tools' help assess the severity of pain, accepting always that it is subjective, and they may also be useful in monitoring the response to treatment. Disturbance of the normal sleep pattern by pain is also useful in

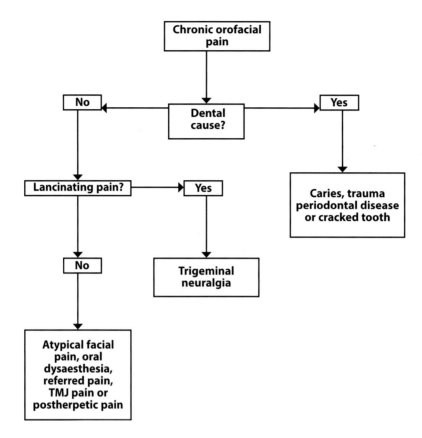

Figure 1. Chronic orofacial pain. (Reproduced from Scully C. *Oral and Maxillofacial Medicine.* Elsevier, 2008.)

assessing the severity.

■ **Duration:** The average duration of each episode may help diagnosis. For example, pain from exposed dentine is fairly transient (lasting only for seconds following application of a stimulus), while the pain from pulpitis lasts for a much longer period. Trigeminal neuralgia is a brief lancinating pain lasting up to about 5 seconds, although some patients report a persistent background less severe pain – more of a dull ache; migrainous neuralgia typically lasts 30–45 minutes, while chronic idiopathic facial pain (atypical facial pain) is typically persistent.

■ **Frequency and periodicity:** Determine whether the pain occurs at specific times or is related to specific events. A 'Pain Diary' can help. For example, the pain of temporomandibular pain dysfunction syndrome may be more severe on waking, if this is associated with nocturnal parafunctional activity such as clenching or tooth grinding. The pain of sinusitis is often aggravated by lying down. Periodic migrainous neuralgia frequently disturbs the patient's sleep at a specific time each night, around 2am. One patient seen by the authors complained of pain fairly typical of periodic migrainous neuralgia, yet appearing

- ■ Reassurance/explanation of the benign and self-limiting nature of the problem;
- ■ Rest (eg soft diet and limitation of movement);
- ■ Anti-inflammatory analgesic (eg ibuprofen 400 mg three times a day);
- ■ Occlusal splint therapy;
- ■ Local physiotherapy.

Table 2. Keypoints: management of TMJ pain-dysfunction.

around 2pm; it turned out he was a long-distance night driver, sleeping mainly during the day!

■ **Precipitating, aggravating and relieving factors:** It may be necessary to resort to leading questions to ask if temperature, biting, posture, analgesics, alcohol, etc affect the pain. For example, heat often aggravates dental pain; touching a trigger zone may precipitate trigeminal neuralgia attacks, stress may worsen atypical facial pain, and alcohol may induce episodes of migrainous neuralgia.

■ **Associated features:** Some types of pain may be associated with other features which are helpful diagnostically, such as the swollen face in dental abscess, nausea and vomiting in migraine, or nasal stuffiness or lacrimation in migrainous neuralgia.

The cause of most orofacial pain is established mainly from the history, and examination findings are also helpful, not least in excluding local pathology. However, it is important to consider the usefulness of a Specialist who can arrange additional investigations, particularly imaging of the head and neck, using CT or MRI. It is crucial not to miss detecting organic disease and thus mislabelling the patient as having psychogenic pain, and not to miss a brain tumour underlying a patient with supposed 'idiopathic' trigeminal neuralgia.

Local causes of orofacial pain

Odontogenic pain

Most orofacial pain is, of course, related to dental disease – odontogenic causes – and will not be described further.

Mucosal pain

Pain from oral mucosal lesions can be either localized or diffuse. Localized pain is usually associated with a mucosal break, either an erosion (a partial thickness loss of epithelium) or ulcer (a full thickness loss of epithelium), discussed in a previous article. Of course, the distinction between these painful conditions can at times be difficult or impossible and many patients have both.

Diffuse pain may also be caused by infection, or a systemic underlying deficiency state or other factors, and is usually then described as 'soreness' or sometimes 'burning'.

Mucosal pain may be aggravated by sour, acidic, spicy, or salty foods, so that few affected patients can tolerate or enjoy citrus fruits or tomatoes for example. The area is usually also tender to touch.

Other local causes of orofacial pain

Jaws

Pain from the jaws can be caused by infection, direct trauma, malignancies, and rarely by Paget's disease. However, unless associated with infection or jaw fracture, retained roots and impacted teeth, and lesions such as cysts, are usually painless.

Malignant tumours usually produce deep, boring pain, sometimes associated with paraesthesia or anaesthesia, but odontogenic and other benign tumours of the bone do not normally produce pain. Lip numbness or tingling, therefore, may herald a tumour in the jaw bone.

- ■ **Rest yourself and your jaw:**
  - ● **Relax and practise stress reduction;**
  - ● **Exercise** regularly;
  - ● **Eat soft foods** and avoid hard, crusty foods like nuts or hard bread or those that need chewing a great deal;
  - ● **Chew on your back teeth,** not the front ones;
  - ● **Eat small bites;**
  - ● **Sleep on your side.**
- ■ **Avoid joint or muscle damage by avoiding:**
  - ● **Contact sports;** wear a mouthguard if you must play contact sports;
  - ● **Excessive jaw use** in yawning, grinding and clenching;
  - ● **Chewing gum;**
  - ● **Habits** such as biting:
    - – Finger nails;
    - – Pens and pencils;
    - – Lip.
  - ● **Excessive mouth-opening in:**
    - – Long dental appointments;
    - – General anaesthesia.
  - ● **Cradling the telephone** between head and shoulder
  - ● **Wind instrument playing**
- ■ **Reduce muscle pain with analgesics and by applying:**
  - ● **Cold packs** for 10 minutes every 3 hours for 72 hours after injury;
  - ● **Hot packs** for 20 minutes every 3 hours to uninjured joints/muscles.
- ■ **Re-educate the jaw opening:**
  - ● **Open your mouth with a hinge movement:** exercise your jaw twice daily, opening 5 times in front of a mirror, ensuring the jaw opens vertically without deviating sideways;
  - ● **Exercise your jaw** 3 times daily for 5 timed minutes:
    - – Close your mouth on the back teeth;
    - – Put the tip of your tongue on the palate behind your front teeth;
    - – Move the tongue back across the palate as far as it will go;
    - – Keep the tongue in this position with the teeth closed for 10 seconds;
    - – Open your mouth slowly until the tongue starts to leave the palate;
    - – Keep that position for 10 seconds;
    - – Close your mouth;
    - – Repeat over 5 minutes.

Table 3. Steps to manage TMJ pain-dysfunction.

	Idiopathic trigeminal neuralgia	Idiopathic facial pain	Migrainous neuralgia
Age (Years)	>50	30–50	30–50
Sex	F>M	F>M	M>F
Site	Unilateral, mandible or maxilla	+ Bilateral, maxilla	Retro-orbital
Associated Features	–	+/– Depression	+/– Conjunctival injection +/– Lacrimation +/– Nasal congestion
Character	Lancinating	Dull	Boring
Duration of episode	Brief (seconds)	Continual	Few hours
Usual timing of pain	Daytime	Daytime	Night-time
Precipitating	Trigger areas	+/– Adverse life events	+/– Alcohol
Main treatments	Carbamazepine	Cognitive behavioural therapy, Antidepressants	Oxygen, sumatriptan

Table 4. Differentiation of important types of chronic orofacial pain.

Salivary glands

Pain from salivary gland disorders is mainly caused by duct obstruction, sometimes by infection or a tumour. The pain is usually localized to the affected gland, may be quite severe, and may be intensified by increased saliva production, such as before and with meals. Examination may reveal a swollen salivary gland, sometimes with tenderness and/or a degree of trismus.

Sinuses and pharynx

Disease of the paranasal sinuses and nasopharynx, which can cause oral and/or facial pain, include sinusitis and tumours, which can remain undetected until they have reached an advanced stage. Any suggestion of

a discharge from the nose, or obstruction to breathing, cheek swelling or numbness or tingling of the upper lip should be taken seriously as they may herald an antral carcinoma.

Pressure on mental nerve

On occasions, if there is dehiscence of the mental nerve, as a result of resorption of the alveolar ridge, pain is caused by pressure from a denture.

Temporomandibular joint pain

Pain from the TMJ may result from dysfunction, trauma, inflammation and, very rarely, tumours, either in the head and neck, or even lungs.

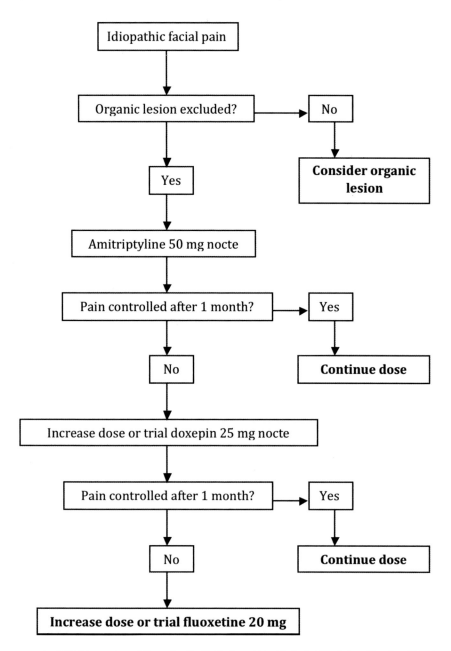

Figure 2. Management of IFP. (Reproduced from Scully C. *Oral and Maxillofacial Medicine.* Elsevier, 2008.)

Temporomandibular pain-dysfunction syndrome

Temporomandibular pain-dysfunction syndrome is a very common problem, characterized by pain, clicking and jaw locking or limitation of opening of the jaw.

Afflicting young women mainly, factors which have been implicated include over-opening of the mouth, muscle overactivity (eg bruxism, clenching), TMJ disruption and psychiatric history (eg anxiety, stressful life events). Precipitating factors may include local trauma, wide mouth opening, or emotional upset.

Diagnosis

Diagnosis is clinical. Pain from TMJ disease is usually dull, poorly localized, may radiate widely, is usually intensified by movement of the mandible and may be associated with trismus because of spasm in the masticatory muscles. Examination may reveal a click from the joint, limited jaw movements, and tender masticatory muscles. Any suggestion of a swollen and/or warm joint suggests true arthritis.

Management

Most patients recover spontaneously and progression to arthritis is virtually unknown. Therefore reassurance and conservative measures are the main management. TMJ pain-dysfunction can usually be effectively managed in general practice. Practitioners are usually well versed with this problem but possible options for treatment in a primary care environment are summarized in Table 2 and patient guidance in Table 3.

Recalcitrant cases may need Specialist attention, particularly if simple measures fail.

Keypoints for patients: temporomandibular (TMJ) pain-dysfunction

- This is a common condition;
- It appears to be related to stress, joint damage or habits involving the teeth and joints (eg tooth clenching or grinding);
- There are no serious long-term consequences; arthritis does not result;
- The symptoms usually clear spontaneously after some months but, in the meantime, rest, exercises, splints, or drugs may help.

Websites and patient information

http://www.aaop.org
http://www.nidcr.nih.gov/OralHealth/Topics/TMJ/TMJDisorders.htm

Psychogenic causes of orofacial pain

Psychogenic (tension) headaches caused by anxiety or stress-induced muscle tension are common, especially in young adults. The pain typically affects the frontal, occipital and/or temporal regions, as a constant ache or band-like pressure, often worse by the evening, but usually abates with rest. Similar problems can affect the orofacial region.

Reassurance may be effective but the pain may also be helped by massage, warmth, non-steroidal anti-

Local causes
– Erythema migrans;
– (geographic tongue);
– Lichen planus;
– Candidosis;
■ Denture problems (eg ill-fitting dentures, inadequate freeway space, encroachment on tongue space);
■ Parafunctional activity (eg tongue thrusting habit, clenching)
Systemic causes
– Psychogenic;
– Cancerophobia;
– Depression;
– Anxiety states;
– Hypochondriasis;
■ Deficiency of:
– Vitamin B, especially B_{12};
– Folate
– Iron
■ Dry mouth
■ Diabetes
■ Drugs

Table 5. Causes of a burning sensation in the mouth.

Medical	Surgical
■ Carbamazepine	■ Cryotherapy
■ Oxcarbazepine	■ Balloon compression of
■ Gabapentin	trigeminal ganglion
■ Lamotrigine	■ Microvascular
	decompression
■ Phenytoin	■ Gamma knife surgery

Table 6. Medical and surgical treatments for ITN.

inflammatory drugs (NSAIDs), or by benzodiazepines, which are both anxiolytic and mild muscle relaxants, or by complementary therapies.

In some studies, nearly 40% of the population have reported frequent headaches and orofacial pain. The reason behind conditions with a psychogenic component, sometimes termed medically unexplained symptoms (MUS), may include:
- Possible links between neuro-humoral mechanisms and altered CNS function;
- The heightening of bodily sensations (lowered pain threshold) as a consequence of physiological processes, such as autonomic arousal, muscle tension, hyperventilation, or inactivity;

■ Misattribution of normal sensations to serious physical disorders.

Features common to most MUS include:
■ Constant chronic discomfort or pain;
■ Pain often of a dull boring or burning type;
■ Pain poorly localized;
■ Pain may cross the mid-line to involve the other side or may move elsewhere;
■ Pain which rarely wakens the patient from sleep;
■ Total lack of objective signs of organic disease;
■ All investigations to identify an underlying organic illness are also negative;
■ There are often recent adverse 'life-events', such as bereavement or family illness;
■ There are often multiple oral and/or other MUS, such as headaches, chronic back or neck pain, pruritus, irritable bowel syndrome, insomnia, numbness or dysmenorrhoea;
■ Cure is uncommon in most, yet few sufferers seem to try to use or persist in using analgesics.

Patients may bring diaries of their symptoms to emphasize their problem. Some have termed this the 'malady of small bits of paper' and, though there is by no means always a psychogenic basis, such notes characterize patients with MUS. These days, this is being replaced by Internet print-outs, which are also increasingly brought by well-informed patients who have no psychogenic problems whatsoever.

Occasional patients quite deliberately induce painful oral lesions and some have Munchausen's syndrome, where they behave in such a fashion as to appear to want operative intervention.

The most common types of orofacial pain with a strong psychogenic component are:
■ Idiopathic (atypical) facial pain;
■ Oral dysaesthesia (burning mouth syndrome);
■ Atypical odontalgia;
■ The syndrome of oral complaints.

Some clinicians also include temporomandibular pain-dysfunction in this category.

Chronic idiopathic facial pain (IFP)

Idiopathic facial pain is a constant chronic orofacial discomfort or pain, defined by the International Headache Society as *facial pain not fulfilling other criteria*. Therefore, like BMS, it is also a diagnosis reached only by the exclusion of organic disease; there are no physical signs, investigations are all negative and it is an MUS. Atypical facial pain is fairly common, affecting probably around 1–2% of the population. Indeed, in some studies, nearly 40% of the population have reported frequent headache and/or orofacial pain.

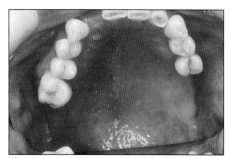
Figure 3. Herpes zoster, palate.

Keypoints: chronic idiopathic facial pain

■ Similar symptoms may be seen in some neurological conditions;
■ Cranial nerve examination should be carried out;
■ X-rays, scans and/or blood tests are often required.

Pain is often of a dull, boring or burning type with an ill-defined location and there is:
■ A total lack of objective signs;
■ A negative result from all investigations;
■ No clear explanation as to cause;
■ Poor response to treatment.

Patients are often middle-aged or older and 70% or more are females. Most sufferers from IFP are otherwise normal individuals who are, or have been, under extreme stress, such as bereavement, or concern about cancer. There are often recent adverse life events, such as bereavement or family illness and/or dental or oral interventional procedures.

Clinical features

History findings in IFP include pain, mainly in the upper jaw, of distribution unrelated to the anatomical distribution of the trigeminal nerve, poorly localized, and sometimes crossing the mid-line to involve the other side or moving to another site. Pain is often of a deep, dull, boring or burning, chronic discomfort, and persists for most or all of the day but does not waken the patient from sleep. However, the patient may report difficulty sleeping.

There may also be multiple oral and/or other psychogenic related complaints, such as dry mouth, bad or altered taste, thirst, headaches, chronic back pain, irritable bowel syndrome or dysmenorrhoea. Patients only uncommonly use analgesics to try to control the pain, but there is a high level of utilization of healthcare services. There have often already been multiple consultations and attempts at treatment.

Pain is accompanied by altered behaviour, anxiety or depression. Over 50% of such patients are depressed or hypochondriacal, and some have lost or been separated from parents in childhood. Many lack insight and will persist in blaming organic diseases (or healthcare professionals) for their pain.

Clinical examination is unremarkable with a total lack of objective physical (including neurological) signs. All imaging studies and blood investigations are negative.

Diagnosis of IFP

Diagnosis is clinical through careful examination of the mouth, peri-oral structures, and cranial nerves, and imaging (tooth/jaw/sinus radiography and MRI/CT scan) to exclude organic disease, such as space-occupying or demyelinating diseases (Table 4).

Management of patients suffering idiopathic facial pain or pain with a psychogenic basis

Few patients with IFP have spontaneous remission and thus treatment is usually indicated (Figure 2).

Reassurance and attention to any factors such as the dentures or haematinic deficiencies may be indicated, but active dental or oral surgical treatment, or attempts at 'hormone replacement', or polypharmacy in the absence of any specific indication, should be avoided.

However, it is important, where possible, to identify and relieve factors which lower the pain threshold (fatigue, anxiety and depression). Simple analgesics such as NSAIDs should be tried initially, before embarking on more potent preparations.

Patient information is a very important aspect in management. Cognitive-behavioural therapy (CBT) or a Specialist referral may be indicated.

It is important to acknowledge clearly the reality of the patient's symptoms and distress and never attempt to trivialize or dismiss them:
■ Try to explain the psychosomatic background to the problem, ascribing the symptoms to causes for which the patient cannot be blamed.
■ Set goals which include helping the patient cope with the symptoms rather than attempting any impossible cure.
■ Do not repeat examinations or investigations at subsequent appointments, since this only serves to reinforce abnormal illness behaviour and health fears.
■ Avoid attempts at relieving pain by operative intervention – since these are rarely successful; indeed, active dental measures such as restorative treatment, endodontics or oral surgical treatment, in the absence of any specific indication, should be avoided as they may simply reinforce the patient's perception that the pain has an organic basis.
■ Offer referral to a Specialist or a trial of antidepressants, explaining that these agents are being used to treat the symptoms not depression, that some antidepressants have analgesic activity, and that antidepressants have been shown in controlled trials to be effective for this problem, even in non-depressed people.

Keypoints for patients: idiopathic facial pain

■ This is fairly common;
■ The cause is not completely known;
■ It may be caused by increased nerve sensitivity;
■ There may be a background of stress;
■ There are usually no serious long-term consequences;
■ X-rays and blood tests *may* be required;
■ Treatment takes time and patience; some nerve-calming drugs can help.

Websites and patient information

http://facial-neuralgia.org/conditions/atfp.html

Burning mouth 'syndrome'(BMS)

There may be definable organic causes of this type of complaint, often described as a burning sensation (Table 5), and a patient in such pain may well also manifest psychological reactions to the experience. However, burning mouth 'syndrome' (BMS: also known as glossopyrosis; glossodynia; oral dysaesthesia; or stomatodynia) is *the term usually used when symptoms, described as a burning sensation, exist in the absence of identifiable organic aetiological factors.* BMS is often a MUS but it must also be recognized that it may well not be a single entity. BMS is a fairly common chronic complaint, affecting up to 0.7–2.6% of the population and seen especially in middle-aged or elderly patients, particularly in females, in a ratio of more than 3:1 and even as high as 7:1. There is no specific relationship to hormonal changes, despite the fact that BMS is often seen in middle-aged or elderly peri- or post-menopausal females. BMS has been reported in 10-40% of women presenting for treatment of menopausal symptoms.

Defined clinical conditions that must be excluded since they can also present with burning include:
■ Erythema migrans (geographic tongue);
■ Lichen planus;
■ Dry mouth;
■ Candidosis;
■ Glossitis such as may be associated with haematinic (iron, folic acid, vitamin B) deficiency;

■ Diabetes.

Uncommon causes that may need to be considered include:
■ Hypothyroidism;
■ Lupus erythematosus;
■ Mucositis;
■ Drugs (especially angiotensin-converting enzyme [ACE] inhibitors; protease inhibitors; cytotoxic agents; clonazepam);
■ Hypersensitivity (to sodium metabisulphite, nuts, dental materials and other substances);
■ Galvanic reactions to metals in the mouth.

Organic problems which sometimes present with no detectable clinical lesions, but that can cause similar symptoms include:
■ A haematological deficiency state (deficiencies in iron, folic acid or vitamin B_{12}) in about 30%;
■ Restricted tongue space from poor denture construction;
■ Parafunction such as nocturnal bruxism or tongue-thrusting;
■ Neuropathy, such as follows damage to the chorda tympani nerve.

No precipitating cause for BMS can be identified in over 50% of the patients but, in others, a psychogenic cause such as anxiety, depression or cancerophobia can be identified in about 20% and, in some patients, BMS appears to follow either dental intervention or an upper respiratory tract infection.

Clinical features

BMS most frequently affects the tongue, but it can also affect the palate or, less commonly, the lips or lower alveolus. The history is that the burning sensation is chronic, usually bilateral, often relieved by eating and drinking, in contrast to pain caused by organic lesions which is typically aggravated by eating. Alcohol may also relieve or reduce the symptoms.

Patients with BMS often have multiple oral and/or other psychogenic related complaints, such as dry mouth, bad or altered taste, thirst, headaches, chronic back pain, irritable bowel syndrome or dysmenorrhoea. There may be changes in sleep patterns and mood and, though patients only uncommonly use analgesics to try to control the symptoms, there have often already been multiple consultations. Interestingly, patients with BMS also have heightened ability to taste – they are 'supertasters'.

Examination shows no clinically detectable signs of mucosal disease or tenderness or swelling of the tongue or affected area, and no neurological or other objective signs.

Keypoints; burning mouth syndrome

■ Similar symptoms may be seen in some organic conditions;
■ Blood tests may be required;
■ Psychological assessment can be helpful.

Diagnosis

Diagnosis of BMS is clinical and it is important to exclude organic causes such as erythema migrans (geographic tongue), candidosis, lichen planus, dry mouth, glossitis, diabetes or denture problems. Importantly, all investigations prove normal.

Investigations indicated may include:
■ Laboratory screening for:

– Anaemia, a vitamin or iron deficiency (blood tests);

– Diabetes (blood and urine analyses);

– Thyroid dysfunction (blood analyses);

– Xerostomia (salivary flow rates);

– Candidosis (oral rinse);

■ Psychological screening using, for example, the Hospital Anxiety and Depression (HAD) scale.

Management is discussed above.

Keypoints for patients: burning mouth syndrome

■ This is a common condition;
■ The cause is not usually known;
■ It may be a nerve hypersensitivity;
■ It is not infectious;
■ It may occasionally be caused by some mouth conditions, dry mouth, deficiencies, diabetes or drugs;
■ It has no long-term consequences;
■ Blood tests or biopsy *may* be required;
■ It may be controlled by some nerve-calming drugs.

Websites and patient information

http://www.go4hope.org
http://www.mayoclinic.com/invoke.
cfm?objectid=4E7AF27F-25B0-43D0-90383E896030B033

Atypical odontalgia

Atypical odontalgia is pain and hypersensitive teeth in the absence of detectable pathology. The pain is typically indistinguishable from pulpitis or periodontitis but is aggravated by dental intervention. Probably a variant of idiopathic facial pain, it should be managed similarly.

The syndrome of oral complaints

Multiple pains and other complaints may occur simultaneously or sequentially, and relief is rarely found (or admitted). Patients may bring diaries of their symptoms to emphasize their problem. This has been termed the 'malady of small bits of paper', and though there is not always a psychogenic basis, such notes characterize patients with non-organic complaints or people with highly obsessional personalities.

Neurological (neuropathic) causes of orofacial pain

Sensory innervation of the mouth, face and scalp depends on the trigeminal nerve, so that diseases affecting this nerve anywhere in the course from the orofacial region to the brain can cause orofacial pain or, indeed, sensory loss, sometimes with serious implications.

Any lesion affecting the trigeminal nerve may cause pain, often with physical signs such as facial sensory or motor impairment. Such causes include:
■ Trauma;
■ Cerebrovascular disease;
■ Demyelinating disease (eg multiple sclerosis);
■ Neoplasia (eg nasopharyngeal, antral or brain tumours); or
■ Infections such as herpes zoster (Figure 3) or HIV/AIDS.

Idiopathic trigeminal neuralgia

Idiopathic trigeminal neuralgia (ITN) is an uncommon nerve disorder that causes episodes of unilateral intense, stabbing, electric shock-like pain in the areas of the face where the branches of the nerve are distributed – lips, eyes, nose, scalp, forehead, upper jaw, or lower jaw. ITN onset is mainly in the 50–70 year age group.

The cause of ITN is unclear, but one hypothesis is that a cerebral blood vessel becomes atherosclerotic and therefore less flexible with age, then pressing on the roots of the trigeminal nerve in the posterior cranial fossa, causing neuronal discharge.

The characteristic features of ITN are summarized as:
A. Paroxysmal attacks of facial or frontal pain which lasts a few seconds to less than 2 minutes. These attacks occur especially in the morning, and rarely cause sleep disturbance.
B. Pain has at least 4 of the following characteristics:
■ Distribution along one or more divisions of the trigeminal nerve;
■ Sudden intense, sharp superficial, stabbing or burning in quality;
■ Pain intensity severe;

■ Precipitation from trigger areas or by certain daily activities such as eating, talking, washing the face, shaving, or cleaning the teeth;
■ Between paroxysms, the patient is usually entirely asymptomatic. Some patients experience a dull ache at other times.
C. No neurological deficit.
D. Attacks are stereotyped in the individual patient.
E. Exclusion of other causes of facial pain by history, physical examination and special investigations when necessary.

A less common form of the disorder called 'Atypical Trigeminal Neuralgia' may cause less intense, constant, dull burning or aching pain, sometimes with occasional electric shock-like stabs. Both forms of the disorder most often affect one side of the face, but some patients experience pain at different times on both sides.

Diagnosis

ITN is universally considered to be one of the most painful afflictions known. Severe pain suggestive of ITN but with physical signs such as facial sensory or motor impairment can result from lesions discussed above. ***These serious conditions must therefore be excluded*** by history, examination; including neurological assessment especially of cranial nerves, and investigations; including imaging (usually MRI) to exclude space-occupying or demyelinating disease, and blood tests to exclude infections and systemic vasculitides.

Only then can the term idiopathic (benign) trigeminal neuralgia be used!

Keypoints; trigeminal neuralgia

■ Similar symptoms may be seen in some neurological conditions;
■ Cranial nerve examination should be carried out;
■ X-rays, scans and/or blood tests are often required.

Management

Few patients with ITN have spontaneous remission and thus treatment is usually indicated. However, ITN is often an intermittent disease with apparent remissions lasting months or years, but recurrence is common and very often the pain spreads to involve a wider area over time and the intervals between episodes tend to shorten.

Patients with supposed ITN are best seen at an early stage by a Specialist in order to confirm the diagnosis and initiate treatment. In the acute situation, the patient's symptoms may be controlled on a short-term basis with injection of a regional local anaesthetic.

Medical treatment, typically using anticonvulsants, is successful for most patients (Table 6). Carbamazepine is the main drug used, but it is not an analgesic and must be given continuously prophylactically for long periods, and under strict medical surveillance. Adverse effects must be monitored, including:
■ Balance (disturbed – ataxia); this tends to be the feature that limits the dose of carbamazepine;
■ Blood pressure (may increase); patients must have a baseline test and then blood pressure estimations for 3 months, then 6-monthly;
■ Blood tests – mainly for liver function (may become impaired); and bone marrow function (red and white cells and/or platelets may be depressed).

Other agents such as gabapentin, phenytoin, lamotrigine and baclofen are available and some patients also report having reduced or relieved pain by means of alternative medical therapies, such as acupuncture, chiropractic adjustment, self-hypnosis or meditation.

Should medical care become ineffective, or produce excessive undesirable side-effects, neurosurgical procedures are available to relieve pressure on the nerve or to reduce nerve sensitivity.

Keypoints for patients: trigeminal neuralgia

■ This is an uncommon disorder;
■ The cause is unknown;
■ It involves spontaneous activity of pain nerves;
■ It is not known to be infectious;
■ Similar symptoms may be seen in some neurological conditions; X-rays, scans and/or blood tests may therefore be required;
■ There are usually no long-term consequences;
■ Symptoms may be controlled with drugs, freezing the nerve, or surgery.

Websites and patient information

http://ihs-classification.org/en/02_klassifikation/04_teil3/13.01.01_facialpain.html
http://www.mayoclinic.com/health/trigeminal-neuralgia/DS00446

Glossopharyngeal neuralgia

Glossopharyngeal neuralgia is much less common than trigeminal neuralgia. Occasionally glossopharyngeal neuralgia is secondary to tumours. The pain is of a similar nature but affects the throat and ear, and typically is triggered by swallowing or coughing. Carbamazepine is usually less effective than for trigeminal neuralgia and adequate relief of pain can be difficult. A Specialist opinion is warranted to investigate and manage these patients.

Herpetic and post-herpetic neuralgia

Herpes zoster (shingles), the recrudescence of herpes-varicella-zoster virus latent in sensory ganglia after chickenpox, is often preceded and accompanied by neuralgia, but a unilateral rash and ulceration is typical (Figure 3). Neuralgia may also persist (post-herpetic neuralgia) after the rash has resolved and can cause continuous burning pain, in contrast to the lancinating pain of trigeminal neuralgia, which also affects mainly elderly patients. A Specialist opinion is warranted to investigate and manage these patients.

Vascular causes of orofacial pain

Several disorders in which the most obvious organic feature is vascular dilatation or constriction can cause orofacial pain. The pain is usually obviously in the face or head rather than in the mouth alone but occasionally can involve both, and can be difficult to differentiate from other causes of orofacial pain (Table 1). These disorders include:
■ Migraine (usually obvious and not causing oral pain alone, and therefore not included here);
■ Migrainous neuralgia;
■ Giant cell arteritis.

Migrainous neuralgia (cluster headache)

Migrainous neuralgia is less common than migraine but more likely to cause orofacial pain. Males are mainly affected (M:F = 4:1) and attacks often begin in about middle age (Table 4). The pain is unilateral, occurs in attacks, is burning and 'boring' in character, and usually localized around the eye. Generally, the attacks commence, and often awaken the patient, at the same time each night or in the early hours of the morning, hence the term 'alarm clock headache'. This pain may be associated with profuse watering and 'congestion' of the conjunctiva, rhinorrhoea and nasal obstruction on the affected side. The attacks usually end in less than one hour. Attacks are sometimes precipitated by alcohol.

Migrainous neuralgia is managed by a Specialist, with a variety of agents, including sumatriptan, beta-blockers, indometacin, or oxygen inhalations.

Cranial arteritis (temporal arteritis; giant-cell arteritis)

Cranial arteritis is a febrile disease, in which giant cells appear in the arteries and cause a deranged internal elastic lamina. It most commonly affects the elderly. The headache is intense, deep and aching, throbbing in nature and persistent. It is frequently made worse when the patient lies flat in bed and it may be exacerbated or reduced by digital pressure on the artery involved. Occasionally, the artery (usually the superficial temporal artery) may be enlarged and tender. It is also characterized by malaise, weakness, weight loss, anorexia, fever, and sweating.

Diagnosis is supported by a raised erythrocyte sedimentation rate and C-reactive protein (or plasma viscosity). Arterial biopsy demonstrates fragmentation of the internal elastic lamina.

Although it is a self-limiting disease, patients with cranial arteritis may be threatened with loss of vision. Accordingly, urgent specialist referral for diagnosis and early treatment with high dose systemic corticosteroids (prednisolone) is indicated.

Referred causes of orofacial pain

Pain may occasionally be referred to the mouth, face or jaws from the following:
■ **Neck**: cervical vertebral disease, especially cervical spondylosis, very occasionally causes pain referred to the face.
■ **Heart**: in patients with angina. The pain usually affects the mandible, is initiated by exercise (especially in the cold) and abates quickly on rest.
■ **Lungs**: orofacial pain emanating from lung cancer is a

well-recognized entity and can mimic, for example, TMJ pain-dysfunction syndrome.
■ **Oesophagus**: pain plus sialorrhoea may result from oesophageal lesions.
■ **Styloid process**: Eagle's syndrome, a rare disorder due to an elongated styloid process (stylalgia), may cause pain on chewing, swallowing or turning the head
■ **Eyes**: pain from the eyes, arising for example, from disorders of refraction, retrobulbar neuritis (eg in multiple sclerosis), or glaucoma, can radiate to the orbit, maxilla or frontal region.
■ **Ears**: middle ear disease may cause headaches or pain in the TMJ region. Conversely, oral disease not infrequently causes pain referred to the ear, particularly from lesions of the posterior tongue.
■ **Pharynx**: carcinoma of the pharynx may cause orofacial pain.

A Specialist opinion is warranted to investigate and manage these patients.

Patients to refer:
■ Trigeminal neuralgia in view of possibility of demyelination or space occupying lesion;
■ Giant cell arteritis in view of risk of blindness;
■ Patients with chronic idiopathic facial pain who need psychological help;
■ Malignancy.

Lumps and Swellings: Neck

10

Neck lumps

The lymphoid system is the essential basis of immune defences and comprises predominantly bone marrow, spleen, thymus and lymph nodes. Tissue fluid drains into lymph nodes which act as 'filters' of antigens and, after processing in the nodes, lymph containing various immunocytes drains from the nodes to lymph ducts and then to the circulation. A lymph node consists of a cortex, paracortex and medulla and is enclosed by a capsule. Lymphocytes and antigens (if present) pass into the node through the afferent lymphatics, are 'filtered', and pass out from the medulla through the efferent lymphatics. The cortex contains B cells aggregated into primary follicles; following stimulation by antigen these develop a focus of active proliferation (germinal centre) and are termed secondary follicles. These follicles are in intimate contact with antigen-presenting dendritic cells. The paracortex contains T cells, and the medulla contains T and B cells.

Causes of lymph node enlargement

Many diseases can present with lesions in the neck but the most common are lesions involving the lymph nodes (Table 1).

Lymph nodes enlarge in oral infections or local infections in the drainage area (virtually anywhere in the head and neck). Most common is an enlarged jugulo-digastric (tonsillar) lymph node, inflamed secondary to a viral upper respiratory tract infection. Children and young adults are predominantly affected (Table 2). Enlarged cervical lymph nodes may also be related to malignant disease in the drainage area (eg carcinoma) or may be a manifestation of systemic disease (eg HIV/AIDS). Adults are predominantly affected.

Examination of cervical lymph nodes

The examination of lymph nodes in the neck is an important part of every orofacial examination. About one-third of all the lymph nodes in the body are in the neck and dental surgeons can often detect serious disease through their examination of the neck.

Inspection of the neck, looking particularly for swellings or sinuses, should be followed by careful palpation of the thyroid gland and all the lymph nodes, searching for swelling or tenderness.

It is prudent to adopt a systematic and methodical approach examining different lymph node groups in turn:
- Submental;
- Submandibular;
- Pre-auricular/parotid;
- Occipital;
- Deep cervical chain.

Both anterior and posterior cervical nodes should be examined as well as other nodes, liver and spleen if systemic disease is a possibility. Most disease in lymph nodes is detected in the anterior triangle of neck, which is bounded superiorly by the mandibular lower border, posteriorly and inferiorly by the sternomastoid muscle, and anteriorly by the midline of the neck. Nodes in this site drain most of the head and neck, except the occiput and back of neck. Lymphadenopathy in the anterior triangle of the neck alone is often due to local disease, especially if the nodes are enlarged on only one side.

A limited number of lymph nodes swell usually because they are involved in an immune response to an infectious agent in the area of drainage and nodes are then often firm, discrete and tender, but are mobile (lymphadenitis). The focus of inflammation can usually be found in the drainage area, which is anywhere on the face, scalp and nasal cavity, sinuses, ears, pharynx and oral cavity. Lymph nodes that are tender may be inflammatory, leukaemia or lymphoma; those that are increasing in size and are hard may be malignant.

Lymph nodes may show reactive hyperplasia to a malignant tumour in the drainage area, or swelling because of metastatic infiltration. The latter may cause the node to feel distinctly hard, and it may become bound down to adjacent tissues ('fixed'), may not be discrete, and may even, in advanced cases, ulcerate through the skin. The neoplasms that frequently metastasize to cervical lymph nodes are oral squamous carcinoma (Article 3), nasopharyngeal carcinoma, tonsillar cancer and thyroid tumours.

Usually one or more anterior cervical nodes are involved, often unilaterally in oral neoplasms anteriorly in the mouth, but otherwise not infrequently bilaterally.

Inflammatory	Infective	Local	Bacterial	Local infections in the head and neck
			Viral	Viral respiratory infections Herpes simplex Herpes zoster Herpangina Rubella
		Systemic	Bacterial	Syphilis Tuberculosis Atypical mycobacterioses Cat scratch fever Brucellosis
			Viral	Glandular fever syndromes (EBV, CMV, HIV, HHV-6)
			Protozoal	Toxoplasmosis
	Probably Infective			Mucocutaneous lymph node syndrome (Kawasaki disease)
	Non-Infective	Sarcoidosis Crohn's disease Connective tissue diseases		
Malignancy	Primary	Leukaemias Lymphomas		
	Secondary	Metastases		
Other	Drugs, eg phenytoin			

Table 1. Causes of cervical lymph node enlargement.

Generalized lymphadenopathy with or without enlargement of other lymphoid tissue, such as liver and spleen (hepatosplenomegaly), suggests a systemic cause.

The local cause may not always be found despite a careful search. For example, children occasionally develop a *Staphylococcus aureus* lymphadenitis (usually in a submandibular node) in the absence of any obvious portal of infection.

More serious is the finding of an enlarged node suspected to be malignant but where the primary neoplasm cannot be found. Nasopharyngeal or tonsillar carcinomas are classic causes of this and an ENT opinion should therefore be

Age	Most common causes of swelling
Child (first decade)	Lymphadenitis due to viral respiratory tract infection
Adolescent and teenager (second decade)	Lymphadenitis due to viral respiratory tract infection; Bacterial infection; Glandular fever syndromes; HIV infection; Toxoplasmosis
Adult (third and fourth decades)	Lymphadenitis; Glandular fever syndromes; HIV infection; Malignancy
After fourth decade	Lymphadenitis; Malignancy

Table 2. Lymph node swellings at different ages. (Reproduced from Scully C. *Oral and Maxillofacial Medicine*. Elsevier, 2008.)

Features	Adolescents and young adults mainly	Sore throat Fever; Lymphadenopathy		
Causal agents	Epstein-Barr virus (EBV)	Cytomegalovirus (CMV)	*Toxoplasma gondii*	Human immune deficiency viruses (HIV)
Investigations	Paul-Bunnell Test EBV antibody titres	CMV antibodies	Sabin-Feldman dye test Specific IgM antibodies T4 (CD4) cell numbers	HIV antibody titres Lymphopenia

Table 3. Glandular fever syndromes.

sought. Clinically unsuspected tonsillar cancer is a common cause of metastasis in a cervical node. Biopsy of the tonsil may reveal a hitherto unsuspected malignancy.

Rare causes of cervical metastases include metastases from stomach or even testicular tumours to lower cervical nodes. However, in some patients with a malignant cervical lymph node, the primary tumour is never located.

Lymph nodes may also swell when there are disorders involving the immune system more generally, such as the glandular fever syndromes, HIV/AIDS and related syndromes, various other viral infections; bacterial infections such as syphilis and tuberculosis; and parasites such as toxoplasmosis. In the systemic infective disorders the nodes are usually firm, discrete, tender and mobile. Lymph nodes may also swell in non-infective lesions such as sarcoidosis, mucocutaneous lymph node syndrome, and neoplasms such as lymphomas and leukaemias (Table 1). In the latter instances, and in the glandular fever syndromes (where there is lymphadenopathy often together with sore throat and fever; Table 3), there is usually enlargement of many or all cervical lymph nodes and in some there is involvement of the whole reticulendothelial system, with generalized lymph node enlargement (detectable clinically in neck, groin and axilla) and enlargement of the liver and spleen (hepatosplenomegaly). In the lymphomas particularly, the nodes may be rubbery, matted together and fixed to deeper structures.

Management

A Specialist opinion is generally indicated.

Lumps and Swellings: Mouth

11

Lumps and swellings: lumps in the mouth

Lumps and swellings in the mouth are common, but of diverse aetiologies (Table 1) and some develop into ulcers, as in various bullous lesions (Article 2) and in malignant neoplasms (Article 3).

Many different conditions, from benign to malignant, may present as oral lumps or swellings (Table 1) including:

Developmental: unerupted teeth, and tori–congenital bony lumps lingual to the mandibular premolars (torus mandibularis; Figure 1), or in the centre of the palate (torus palatinus; Figure 2) are common causes of swellings related to the jaws (Article 13).

Inflammatory: dental abscess is one of the most common causes of oral swelling. However, there is a group of conditions characterized by *chronic* inflammation and granulomas, which can present with lumps or swellings. These, include Crohn's disease, orofacial granulomatosis (OFG), and sarcoidosis, which are discussed below.

Traumatic: haematoma may cause a swelling at the site of trauma. The flange of a denture impinging on the vestibular mucosa may stimulate a reactive irregular hyperplasia (denture-induced hyperplasia) (Figure 3).

Neoplasms: benign epulides (Figure 4), fibrous lumps (Figure 5) or malignant tumours such as oral squamous cell carcinoma (OSCC), Kaposi's sarcoma and other neoplasms may present as swellings, as discussed in Article 3. Occasionally, metastatic malignant disease may present as a lump.

Fibro-osseous lesions: fibrous dysplasia and Paget's disease can result in hard jaw swellings.

Hormonal and metabolic: pregnancy may result in a gingival swelling (pregnancy epulis).

Drug-induced: a range of drugs can produce gingival swelling – most common are phenytoin, calcium channel blockers and ciclosporin (Figure 6).

Allergic lesions: angioedema in particular can cause swellings.

Viral lesions: papillomas, common warts (verruca vulgaris) and genital warts (condyloma acuminatum) are all among the lumps caused by human papillomaviruses (HPV; Figure 7).

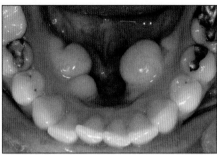
Figure 1. Mandibular tori.

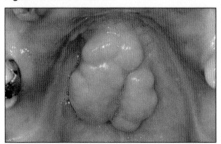
Figure 2. Palatal torus.

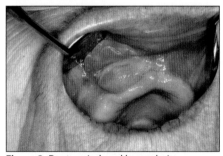
Figure 3. Denture-induced hyperplasia.

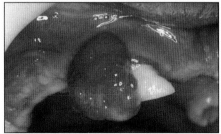
Figure 4. Epulis.

Causes of lumps and swellings according to site

Carcinomas and other malignant neoplasms (Article 3) and pyogenic granulomas (Figure 8) can present in any site.

Gingiva

Sometimes, hyperplasia is congenital. Rapidly developing localized lumps, usually associated with discomfort, are most likely to be abscesses, usually a dental abscess. Other localized swellings are usually inflammatory, such as the pyogenic granuloma, or neoplastic.

Most generalized gingival swellings are due to hyperplasia with oedema related to plaque deposits, occasionally exacerbated by hormonal changes (puberty, pregnancy) or drugs. Such changes often develop slowly – over weeks rather than days – and are usually without discomfort.

There are very few serious causes of generalized enlargements of the gingivae appearing spontaneously or rapidly, but leukaemia is a prime example.

Palate

Lumps of the hard palate may develop from structures within the palate (intrinsic) or beyond it (extrinsic). Thus, for example, torus palatinus is an intrinsic bone lesion, whereas a dental abscess pointing on the palate (usually from the palatal roots of the first and second maxillary molars, or from upper lateral incisors) is extrinsic. Unerupted teeth, especially permanent canines, or second premolars are relatively common. Other causes of palatal swellings are uncommon but it should be remembered that the palate is the second most common site (after the parotid) for pleomorphic adenomas and other salivary neoplasms. Invasive carcinoma from the maxillary sinus may produce a palatal swelling. Kaposi's sarcoma, typical of HIV/AIDS, may also present as a lump in the palate, or elsewhere. Developing unilateral hard palatal swellings, characteristically disturbing the fit of an upper denture in older patients, may denote Paget's disease.

Floor of mouth

Swellings in the floor of the mouth are more likely to arise from structures above the mylohyoid muscle than below it. The commonest swellings in the floor of the mouth are denture-induced hyperplasia and a salivary calculus.

Other lesions producing swellings in this area are a mucocele arising from the sublingual salivary gland (known as ranula because of the resemblance to a frog's belly) and neoplasms of the sublingual salivary gland (usually

Normal Anatomy	Pterygoid hamulus Parotid papillae Lingual papillae
Developmental	Unerupted teeth Odontogenic cysts Eruption cysts Developmental cysts (eg thyroglossal, dermoid) Haemangioma Lymphangioma Maxillary and mandibular tori Hereditary gingival fibromatosis Lingual thyroid
Inflammatory	Abscess Cellulitis Cysts Sialadenitis Pyogenic granuloma Chronic granulomatous disorders – Orofacial granulomatosis – Crohn's disease – Sarcoidosis Insect bites
Traumatic	Denture-induced hyperplasia Epulis Fibro-epithelial polyp Haematoma Mucocele Surgical emphysema
Neoplasms	Carcinoma Leukaemia Lymphoma Myeloma Odontogenic tumours Minor salivary gland tumours Others
Fibro-osseous	Cherubism Fibrous dysplasia Paget's disease
Hormonal	Pregnancy epulis/gingivitis Oral contraceptive pill gingivitis
Metabolic	Amyloidosis Other deposits
Drugs	Phenytoin Calcium channel blockers Ciclosporin
Allergic	Angioedema
Infective	HPV

Table 1. Main conditions which may present as lumps or swellings in the mouth.

malignant), but these are relatively uncommon. Patients occasionally describe a lump which proves to be a swelling of the lingual aspect of the mandible (more characteristic of ameloblastoma than of dental abscesses or cysts). Swellings of the submandibular salivary gland and adjacent lymph nodes may occasionally be described by patients as being in the floor of the mouth. However, only very large swellings below the mylohyoid muscle are likely to produce a bulge in the mouth. Swellings in the floor of the mouth may inhibit swallowing and have an effect on speech.

Mandibular tori produce bony hard swellings lingual to the lower premolars.

Tongue and buccal mucosa

Discrete lumps may be of various causes – congenital (Figure 9; haemangioma), inflammatory, traumatic or neoplastic.

The tongue may be congenitally enlarged (macroglossia) in, for example, Down's syndrome, or may enlarge in angioedema, gigantism, acromegaly or amyloidosis.

Causes of swellings include haematomas from trauma (such as occasional biting), infections, angioedema, fibro-epithelial polyps, fibrous lumps, mucoceles, vesiculobullous lesions and, occasionally, insect bites.

Systemic conditions such as Crohn's disease, orofacial granulomatosis and, occasionally, sarcoid may produce lip swelling (Figure 10) or widespread irregular thickening (cobble-stoning) of the cheek mucosa (Figure 11).

Some 'lumps' become ulcers, as in various bullous lesions, in primary and tertiary syphilis and in malignant neoplasms.

The flange of a denture impinging on the vestibular mucosa may stimulate a reactive irregular hyperplasia – the so-called denture granuloma or denture-induced hyperplasia. Salivary neoplasms in the lip may simulate, but are usually harder than, mucous cysts. Mucoceles are uncommon in the upper lip; discrete swellings there may well be a salivary gland neoplasm.

Diagnosis of the cause of a lump or swelling

When patients refer to a lump in the mouth it is important to establish when it was first noticed. The tongue often detects even very small swellings and patients may also notice a lump because it is sore. Most patients have only a passing interest in their mouths but some examine their mouths out of idle curiosity, some through fear (perhaps after hearing of someone with 'mouth cancer'). Indeed, it is not unknown for some individuals (including dentists!) to discover and worry about the parotid papilla, foliate

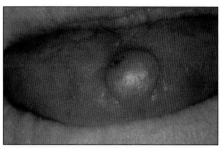
Figure 5. Fibrous overgrowth.

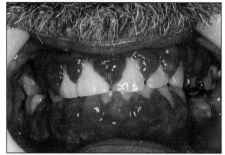
Figure 6. Calcium channel blocker-induced gingival swelling.

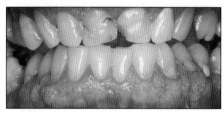
Figure 7. Human papillomavirus infection.

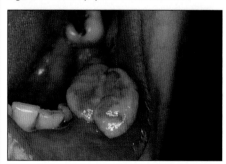
Figure 8. Pyogenic granuloma.

papillae on the tongue, or the pterygoid hamulus. The medical history should be fully reviewed, and there should be a thorough examination, since some systemic disorders, such as neurofibromatosis (Figures 12 and 13), may be associated with intra-oral or facial swellings.

Features of a lump which can be diagnostically useful are:

■ The number of lesions, particularly with regard to whether the lesion is bilaterally symmetrical and thus possibly anatomical;
■ Alteration in size;
■ Any discharge from the lesion (clear fluid, pus, blood);
■ Duration.

Important features to consider when making the provisional diagnosis of the cause of a lump or swelling include:
■ **Position.** The anatomical position should be defined and the proximity to other structures (eg teeth) noted:
– Midline lesions tend to be developmental in origin (eg torus palatinus);
– Bilateral lesions tend to be benign (eg sialosis – salivary swelling in alcoholism, diabetes or other conditions);
– Most neoplastic lumps are unilateral.

Other similar or relevant changes elsewhere in the oral cavity should be noted:
■ **Size**. The size should always be measured and recorded. A diagram or photograph may be helpful.
■ **Shape**. Some swellings have a characteristic shape which may suggest the diagnosis: thus a parotid swelling often fills the space between the posterior border of the mandible and the mastoid process.
■ **Colour**. Brown or black pigmentation may be due to a variety of causes such as a tattoo, naevus or melanoma. Purple or red may be due to a haemangioma, Kaposi's sarcoma or giant cell lesion.
■ **Temperature**.The skin overlying acute inflammatory lesions, such as an abscess, or a haemangioma, is frequently warm.
■ **Tenderness**. Inflammatory swellings such as an abscess are characteristically tender, although clearly palpation must be gentle to avoid excessive discomfort to the patient.
■ **Discharge.** Note any discharge from the lesion (eg clear fluid, pus, or blood), orifice, or sinus.
■ **Movement**. The swelling should be tested to determine if it is fixed to adjacent structures or the overlying skin/mucosa such as may be seen with a neoplasm.
■ **Consistency**. Palpation showing a hard (indurated) consistency may suggest a carcinoma. Palpation may cause the release of fluid (eg pus from an abscess) or cause the lesion to blanch (vascular), or occasionally cause a blister to appear (Nikolsky sign) or to expand. Sometimes palpation causes the patient pain (suggesting an inflammatory lesion). The swelling overlying a bony cyst may crackle (like an egg-shell) when palpated or fluctuation may be elicited by detecting movement of fluid when the swelling is compressed. Palpation may disclose an underlying structure (eg the crown of a tooth under an eruption cyst) or show that the actual swelling is in deeper structures (eg submandibular calculus).
■ **Surface texture**. The surface characteristics should

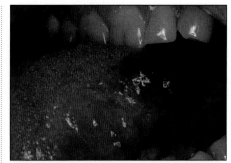

Figure 9. Vascular hamartoma (haemangioma).

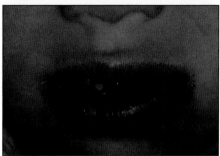

Figure 10. Orofacial granulomatosis.

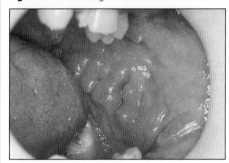

Figure 11. Cobble-stoning of buccal mucosa.

be noted: papillomas have an obvious anemone-like appearance; carcinomas and other malignant lesions tend to have a nodular surface and may ulcerate. Abnormal blood vessels suggest a neoplasm.
■ **Ulceration**. Some swellings may develop superficial ulceration such as squamous cell carcinoma. The character of the edge of the ulcer and the appearance of the ulcer base should also be recorded.
■ **Margin**. Ill-defined margins are frequently associated with malignancy, whereas clearly defined margins are suggestive of a benign lesion.
■ **Number of swellings**. Multiple lesions suggest an infective or occasionally developmental, origin. Some conditions are associated with multiple swellings of a similar nature, eg neurofibromatosis.

Investigations

The nature of many lumps cannot be established without further investigation.
- Any teeth adjacent to a lump involving the jaw should be tested for vitality, and any caries or suspect restorations investigated.
- The periodontal status of any involved teeth should also be determined.
- Imaging of the full extent of the lesion and possibly other areas is required whenever lumps involve the jaws. OPT and special radiographs (eg of the skull, sinuses, salivary gland function), computerized tomography (CT scans) or magnetic resonance imaging (MRI), or ultrasound may, on occasions, be indicated. Photographs may be useful for future comparison.
- Blood tests may be needed, particularly if there is suspicion that a blood dyscrasia or endocrinopathy may underlie the development of a lump.
- Biopsy is often required, especially if the lesion is single and chronic, since it may be a neoplasm or other serious condition.

Chronic granulomatous conditions

There are a number of conditions which present as chronic swellings or lumps, and on biopsy have histological evidence of non-caseating epithelioid cell granulomas. These conditions include orofacial granulomatous, Crohn's disease, and sarcoidosis.

Orofacial granulomatosis

Orofacial granulomatosis (OFG) is an uncommon but increasingly recognized condition, seen mainly in adolescents and young adults, which usually manifests with facial and/or labial swelling, but which can also manifest with angular stomatitis and/or cracked lips, ulcers, mucosal tags, cobble-stoning or gingival swelling (Figures 10, 11;
Table 2).

Some patients with similar features have, or develop, gastrointestinal Crohn's disease or sarcoidosis.

The aetiology of OFG is unknown but in some there is a postulated reaction to food or other antigens (particularly to additives/preservatives such as benzoates or cinnamaldehyde), or metals such as cobalt. Most patients appear to develop the problem in relation to dietary components such as chocolate, nuts, cheese or food additives.

Conditions related to OFG include Miescher cheilitis, where lip swelling is seen in isolation, and Melkersson-Rosenthal syndrome, where there is facial swelling with fissured tongue and recurrent facial palsy.

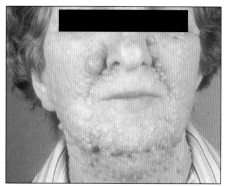
Figure 12. Neurofibromatosis, face.

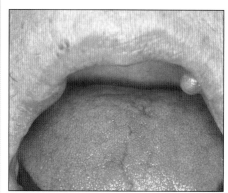
Figure 13. Neurofibromatosis, upper lip.

- Ulcers;
- Facial or labial swelling;
- Lip fissures;
- Mucosal tags;.
- 'Cobble-stone' proliferation of the mucosa;
- Gingival swelling and full-width granular gingivitis.

Table 2. Main features of OFG.

Diagnosis

Diagnosis is clinical, supported by blood tests, endoscopy, imaging and biopsy to differentiate from Crohn's disease, sarcoidosis, tuberculosis and foreign body reactions. Specialist care is usually indicated.

Management

Management is to eliminate allergens such as chocolate, nuts, cheese, cinnamaldehyde or food additives and treat lesions with intralesional corticosteroids or occasionally systemic clofazimine or sulfasalazine.

Useful websites

http://www.emedicine.com/derm/topic72.htm

Crohn's disease

Crohn's disease is a chronic inflammatory idiopathic granulomatous disorder. Many causal factors have been hypothesized but not proved. Crohn's disease affects mainly the small intestine (ileum) but can affect any part of the gastrointestinal tract, including the mouth.

About 10% of patients with Crohn's disease of the bowel have oral lesions. Oral lesions may be seen in the absence of any identifiable gut involvement and are the same as those seen in OFG – reddish raised lesions on the gingiva, hyperplastic folds of the oral mucosa (thickening and folding of the mucosa producing a 'cobble-stone type' of appearance, and mucosal tags), ulcers (classically linear vestibular ulcers with flanking granulomatous masses), facial swelling and angular cheilitis. There may also be features of gastrointestinal involvement, such as abnormal bowel movements, abdominal pain, rectal bleeding or weight loss.

Diagnosis

Oral biopsy, haematological, gastrointestinal and other investigations may be required in suspected Crohn's disease especially to exclude sarcoidosis. Specialist care is usually indicated. Histologically, the epithelium is
intact but thickened, with epithelioid cells and giant cells surrounded by a lymphocytic infiltration.

Management

Topical or intralesional corticosteroids may effectively control the oral lesions but more frequently systemic corticosteroids, azathioprine or salazopyrine are required.

Sarcoidosis

Sarcoidosis is a multi-system granulomatous disorder, of unclear aetiology, which most commonly affects young adult females, especially Afro-Caribbeans.

Sarcoidosis typically causes bilateral hilar lymphadenopathy, pulmonary infiltration and impaired respiratory efficiency, skin and eye lesions, but can involve virtually any tissue. Because of its vague and protean manifestations, sarcoidosis appears to be under-diagnosed. Gingival enlargement, or oral swellings may be seen but sarcoidosis can involve any of the oral tissues and has a predilection for salivary glands, causing asymptomatic enlargement of the major salivary glands and some have xerostomia. The association of salivary and lacrimal gland enlargement with fever and uveitis is known as uveoparotid fever (Heerfordt's syndrome).

Diagnosis

The most helpful investigations include:
■ Chest radiography (for enlarged hilar lymph nodes);
■ Raised levels of serum angiotensin-converting enzyme (SACE) in acute disease;
■ A positive gallium or PET scan of lacrimal and salivary glands;
■ Labial salivary gland biopsy (for histological evidence of non-caseating epithelioid cell granulomas).

Management

Patients with sarcoidosis but only minor symptoms often require no treatment. If there is active ocular disease, progressive lung disease, hypercalcaemia, or cerebral involvement or other serious complications, corticosteroids are given.

Patients to refer:
■ Suspected malignancy in neck including lymphoma;
■ Suspected metastatic disease in neck;
■ Unexplained lymphadenopathy.

Lumps and Swellings: Salivary

12

Salivary gland swelling

Salivary glands usually swell because of inflammation (sialadenitis) (Figure 1), which is often viral but may have other causes (Table 1). Obstruction of salivary flow is another common cause (obstructive sialadenitis) (Figures 2, 3). Rare causes include salivary gland or other neoplasms (Figures 4–7).

In children, most salivary gland swellings are caused by mucoceles or mumps. In adults, most swellings of the salivary glands are caused by mucoceles (Figure 8), salivary duct obstruction (typically by a stone); but sialadenitis,

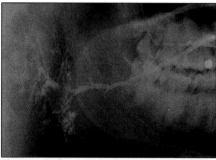

Figure 1. Right parotid sialogram showing dilation of the intraglandular ducts consistent with sialadenitis.

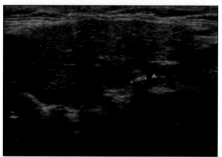

Figure 2. Ultrasound of submandibular gland, stone identified (A).

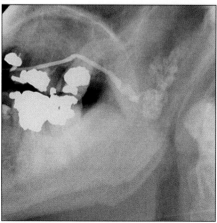

Figure 3. Left parotid sialogram showing intraglandular ductal dilation and a filling defect at the hilum of the gland consistent with a parotid calculus.

- ■ Inflammatory
    - – Mucoceles
    - – Mumps
    - – Ascending sialadenitis
    - – Recurrent parotitis of childhood
    - – HIV parotitis
    - – Other infections (eg tuberculosis)
    - – Sjögren's syndrome
    - – Sarcoidosis
    - – Cystic fibrosis
- ■ Neoplasms (mainly pleomorphic salivary adenoma, but also monomorphic adenomas and malignant tumours)
- ■ Duct obstruction (eg calculus)
- ■ Sialosis (usually caused by autonomic dysfunction in starvation, bulimia, diabetes, or alcoholic cirrhosis)
- ■ Deposits rarely (eg amyloidosis and haemochromatosis)
- ■ Drugs rarely (eg chlorhexidine, methyl dopa, phenylbutazone, iodine compounds, thiouracil, catecholamines, sulfonamides, phenothiazines and protease inhibitors

Table 1. Causes of salivary gland swelling.

Sjögren's syndrome and neoplasms are important causes to be excluded.

Diagnosis of salivary gland swelling

It can be difficult to establish whether a major salivary gland is genuinely swollen, especially in obese patients. A useful guide to whether the patient is simply obese or has parotid enlargement is to observe the outward deflection of the ear lobe, which is seen in true parotid swelling.

Diagnosis of the cause is mainly clinical but investigations such as imaging (especially ultrasound), liver function tests, serology for viral antibodies autoantibodies or biopsy, may be indicated.

Management

A specialist opinion is usually needed and treatment is of the underlying cause.

Immediate treatment is needed for acute bacterial sialadenitis; under ideal conditions antimicrobial therapy should be determined by results of culture and sensitivity of a sample of pus from the duct. However, as first line therapy a penicillinase-resistant penicillin such as flucloxacillin is appropriate. In patients with penicillin allergy, erythromycin is a suitable alternative. In addition, general supportive measures such as analgesia and increased fluid intake are important. Thereafter, specialist referral is generally indicated to identify any predisposing factors. Neoplasms need Specialist attention.

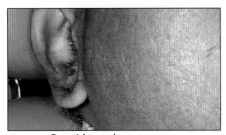

Figure 4. Parotid neoplasm.

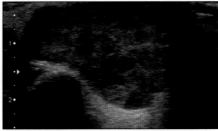

Figure 5. Well defined area of hypo-echogenicity within salivary tissue consistent with a parotid neoplasm.

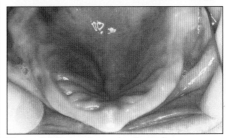

Figure 6. Minor salivary gland neoplasm.

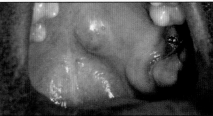

Figure 7. Malignant salivary gland neoplasm.

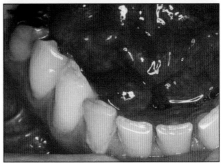

Figure 8. Mucocele, floor of mouth (ranula).

Lumps and Swellings: Jaws

13

Disorders in the jaws

Many diseases of, or in, the jaws present asymptomatically, as *radiolucencies*, *radio-opacities* or with mixed appearances on radiographs. Other presentations are as *swellings, pain* or sometimes *fracture* or *disturbance of tooth eruption* (displaced, missing or loose teeth). Swellings that appear to originate from the jaws may arise from subcutaneous tissues or bones. The mnemonic MINT aids diagnosis:

Malformations, eg tori and fibro-osseous lesions.

Inflammatory conditions, eg odontogenic infections, osteomyelitis, actinomycosis, tuberculosis, or syphilis.

Neoplasms and cysts (see below).

Trauma causing subperiosteal haematomas.

Investigations largely involve imaging, and serum calcium, phosphate, and alkaline phosphatase levels but histopathology is almost invariably required.

Pseudo-diseases

Some jaw conditions are 'pseudo-diseases', including: unerupted teeth, tori (Figures 1–3), bone marrow defects, traumatic bone cyst, Stafne bone defect (static bone cyst), osteosclerosis, pseudocyst of maxillary sinus, or sub-pontic osseous hyperplasia.

A number of bone diseases may also affect the jaws.

Non-neoplastic diseases

- *Arteriovenous malformations.*
- *Central giant cell lesion.*
- *Fibro-osseous lesions.*
- *Infections* (eg osteomyelitis).
- *Metabolic bone disorders* (eg osteomalacia, hyperparathyroidism).
- *Osteonecrosis.* Osteoradionecrosis (ORN) and bisphosphonate-related osteochemonecrosis of the jaws (BRONJ) are uncommon complications of radiation therapy of head and neck tumours, and bisphosphonate

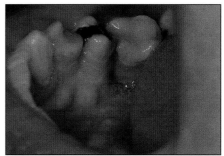
Figure 1. Torus mandibularis.

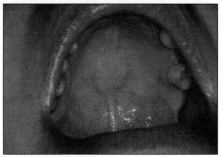
Figure 2. Torus palatinus.

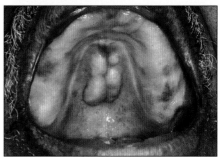
Figure 3. Torus palatinus.

use (especially when given intravenously), respectively. The bone repair response is impaired by these therapies, and surgical interventions (eg tooth extraction) may precipitate the osteonecrosis. Early findings on DPT and CT are sclerosis commonly affecting the alveolar margin, thickening of lamina dura and poor healing or non-healing of extraction sockets. When established, osteonecrosis can be demonstrated on plain radiography and CT as mixed sclerosis and lysis, sequestra, bone fragmentation, soft-tissue swelling and pathological fracture.

■ *Osteopetrosis.* A rare syndrome caused by osteoclast defects, this presents with excessive bone calcification, causing a marble like radio-opacity of the skeleton, and multiple fractures. Complications may also include jaw osteomyelitis, especially in the mandible (in 10%), anaemia, hepatomegaly, and cranial nerve compression. Investigations include radiography and blood tests (low blood calcium, and often raised serum phosphatase). Management with vitamin D (calcitriol), gamma interferon, erythropoietin and corticosteroids may help.

Neoplastic disorders

■ *Bone neoplasms* (Table 1).
■ *Ewing sarcoma.* This is a rare malignant round-cell tumour of young males mainly, affecting bones and soft tissues, presenting as a radiolucent lesion with a lamellated or 'onion skin' type of periosteal reaction. It is positive for CD99 (**C**luster of **D**ifferentiation 99) marker. As many as 30% have metastasized by the time of presentation. Chemotherapy gives a five-year survival for localized disease up to 80% but only one third of this if metastasized.
■ *Langerhans' cell histiocytoses* (LCH) or granulomatosis. Histocytic disorders are divided into:
(1) dendritic cell histiocytosis;
(2) erythrophagocytic macrophage disorders; and
(3) malignant histiocytosis.

LCH belongs in the first group and encompasses a number of rare diseases associated with a reactive increase in bone marrow-derived Langerhans cells (histiocytes – activated dendritic cells and macrophages) in the bone marrow, and sometimes in skin and other organs, they can behave like malignant diseases. Major categories include:

- *Eosinophilic granuloma.* Solitary, indolent and chronic, bone involvement.
- *Hand-Schuller-Christian disease.* An intermediate form with multiple bone involvement, with

Benign	Malignant
Chondroma	Chrondrosarcoma
Osteoblastoma	Osteosarcoma
Osteochondroma	
Osteoma	

Table 1. Bone neoplasms.

■ Cemento-osseous dysplasia
■ Cherubism
■ Fibrous dyplasia
■ Hypercementosis
■ Ossifying fibroma
■ Paget's disease of bone

Table 2. Fibro-osseous dysplasia.

or without skin involvement, characterized by multifocal, chronic involvement – classically the triad of diabetes insipidus, proptosis and lytic bone lesions.
- *Letterer-Siwe disease.* Acute fulminant, disseminated multiple organ involvement with bone and liver lesions.

■ *Leukaemias.* Any of the five leukocyte types can be affected by malignant change-leukaemia. The malignant leukocytes are dysfunctional (predisposing the patient to infections), and crowd other cells out of the bone marrow, so that frequently not enough normal blood cells are made. This leads to anaemia, because red cell production is

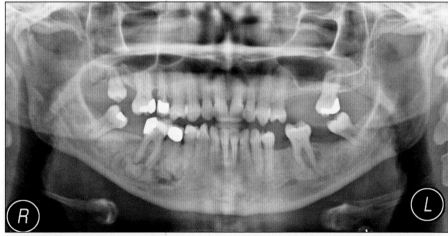

Figure 4. Osseous dysplasia florid type. DPT showing multiple periapical radiolucencies with central opacities of similar density to bone/cementum. Teeth vital.

impaired, and to excessive bleeding and bruising as platelets are impaired. Patients with leukaemia present therefore with anaemia, bruising and bleeding and liability to infections. Jaw involvement may include pain and swelling, or sensory disturbances. Imaging may confirm osteolytic lesions; expanded, coarse marrow spaces and trabeculae; alveolar bone destruction; loss of lamina dura and border of developmental dental crypts; and a periosteal reaction with an 'onion skin' effect.

- *Myelodysplastic Syndrome* (MDS). Diseases also characterized by abnormal bone marrow cell production and not enough normal blood cells are made, leading to anaemia, infection, excessive bleeding and bruising. MDS are, in essence, pre-leukaemia and leukaemia may result.
- *Myeloproliferative disorders* (MPD). Diseases characterized by overproduction of precursor (immature form) marrow cells.
- *Aplastic anaemia*. Associated with loss of cell precursors (usually erythrocytes) due to stem cell defects or injuries to the marrow environment.
- *Lymphomas*. Malignant diseases of lymphocytes, lymphomas and other cancers that spread into the bone marrow can affect cell production. Clinical presentation includes ill-defined radiolucencies in bone.
- *Metastases*. The most frequent sites of primary neoplasms resulting in metastases are kidney, lung, breast, colon, prostate and stomach. Metastases to the jaws are rare, usually to the posterior mandible, and typically manifest with pain and swelling, or sensory disturbances. Not uncommon are loosening of teeth, pathologic jaw fracture, or intraosseous lesions with lytic, ill-defined radiolucencies.
- *Plasma cell disorders*. These conditions (eg multiple myeloma) associated with overproduction of a B lymphocyte clone and its antibody, may affect the jaws. Radiographic findings include: sharply defined radiolucencies, usually of many bones; absence of marginal hyperostosis or opaque lining.

Fibro-osseous lesions

Fibro-osseous lesions are a group of conditions characterized by replacement of normal bone by a proliferating fibrous stroma which forms varying amounts of woven bone spicules and cementum-like material (Table 2).

Cemento-osseous dysplasia

Cemento-osseous dysplasia (COD), periapical cemental or cemento-osseous dysplasia (PCD) or cementoma is an older term)

Cemento-osseous dysplasia is a fibro-osseous lesion common in black females during fourth and fifth decades,

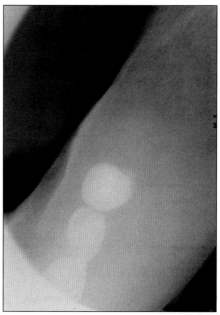

Figure 5. Lower occlusal view showing expansion of the mandible with loss of corticomedullary differentiation and a homogeneous bone pattern (ground glass) associated with fibrous dysplasia.

presenting with radiolucent and radio-opaque lesions at the apices of vital teeth (periapical type), which may be isolated (focal) or multi-quadrant (florid) (Figure 4). Lesions usually involve the mandibular anterior teeth, start as well-circumscribed radiolucent lesions and progressively become radio-opaque centrally, although a thin radiolucent margin is usually visible (helpful in distinguishing from enostosis [idiopathic osteosclerosis]). The lesions are asymptomatic, usually incidental radiographic findings, and the related teeth are vital. Florid COD is probably a widespread form, also occurring mainly in black females but usually affecting three or four quadrants. Bone expansion may occur, and the lesions may present with pain. Bone cysts may develop, and there is a liability to osteomyelitis. Sometimes COD occurs as isolated lesions unassociated with teeth (focal cemento-osseous dysplasia).

COD is self-limiting, so treatment is best limited to symptomatic relief of active infection and localized sequestration. In some cases of florid COD, surgical removal may be required.

Cherubism

The name for this comes from the appearance of angelic putti (chubby boys) in Renaissance art, misnamed by some as cherubs. The mandible in particular is replaced with excessive fibrous tissue which usually resolves as the child matures. Rarely it causes premature loss of primary and uneruption of permanent teeth. Though sometimes named familial fibrous dysplasia of the jaws, cherubism is an autosomal dominant condition involving the SH3BP2 gene and has little in common with fibrous dysplasia.

Fibrous dysplasia

Fibrous dysplasia (FD) is a self-limiting, fibro-osseous lesion caused by mutation in the gene encoding G protein (GNAS1). FD usually affects only one bone (monostotic: about 70%) but occasionally several bones (polyostotic). Maxillofacial fibrous dysplasia may occur anywhere in the jaws but is essentially monostotic and typically affects the maxilla in young people, although it sometimes affects adjacent bones (*craniofacial fibrous dysplasia*), but rarely crosses the midline. CT can best assess the extent in the facial skeleton.

McCune-Albright's syndrome is FD bone lesions with skin pigmentation and endocrinopathy (precocious puberty in females and hyperthyroidism in males).

Bone enlarges in FD but the morphology is preserved, distinguishing FD from a neoplasm. FD lesions vary from radiolucent to radio-opaque, often a 'ground-glass appearance' (Figure 5) with ill-defined margins – a feature helpful to distinguish it from other lesions. Typically, no treatment is needed. Bisphosphonates can help and surgery may be indicated if there is major deformity or pressure on nerves.

Hypercementosis

Hypercementosis is increased deposition of cementum on roots, caused by local trauma, inflammation, Paget's disease, or may occur idiopathically.

Ossifying fibroma (Cemento-ossifying fibroma)

Ossifying fibroma is a usually benign, slow-growing, painless bone neoplasm, typically monostotic and seen in the third and fourth decades in the posterior mandible as a radiolucent, radio-opaque, or mixed opacity and which has a fibro-osseous microscopic appearance. Ossifying fibroma and focal COD are not easily differentiated histopathologically. Juvenile ossifying fibroma is an aggressive variant with a rapid growth pattern seen mainly in boys aged under 15 years.

Traditionally, the initial treatment has been simple curettage. More definitive resection has been reserved for recurrent disease.

Paget's disease of bone

Paget's disease of bone (PDB) is a progressive fibro-osseous disease affecting bone and cementum, characterized by disorganization of osteoclastogenesis (osteoclast formation) – a process dependent on two cytokines, macrophage colony stimulating factor (M-CSF) and receptor activator of nuclear factor kappa-B ligand (RANKL), which induce gene expression changes, presumably by inducing transcription factors. The tumour necrosis factor (TNF) receptor superfamily activate nuclear factor kappa-B (NF-κB), and RANK (for receptor activator of NF- kappa B), which is involved in osteoclastogenesis.

Seen mainly in males over 55 years of age, there is a strong genetic component; 15–20% have a first-degree relative with PDB. Genes involved include the sequestosome1 gene (SQSTM1).

In PDB, bone remodelling is disrupted, and an anarchic alternation of bone resorption and apposition results in mosaic-like 'reversal lines'. Most patients are asymptomatic. A minority of patients with Paget's disease experience a variety of symptoms, including bone pain secondary osteoarthritis, bone deformity and neurological complications due to compression of nerves.

In early lesions, bone destruction predominates (osteolytic stage) and there is bowing of the long bones, especially the tibia, pathological fractures, broadening/flattening of the chest and spinal deformity. The increased bone vascularity can lead to high output cardiac failure.

Later, as disease activity declines, bone apposition increases (osteosclerotic stage) and bones enlarge, with progressive thickening (between these phases is a mixed phase). PDB is typically polyostotic and may affect skull, skull base, sphenoid, orbital and frontal bones. The maxilla often enlarges, particularly in the molar region, with widening of the alveolar ridge. In early lesions, large irregular areas of relative radiolucency (osteoporosis circumscripta) are seen, but later there is increased radio-opacity, with appearance of 'cotton wool' pattern. Constriction of skull foramina may cause cranial neuropathies. The dense bone and hypercementosis makes tooth extraction difficult, and there is also a liability to haemorrhage and infection.

Diagnosis supported by imaging, biochemistry and histopathology. Bone scintiscanning shows localized areas of high uptake. Plasma alkaline phosphatase and urine hydroxyproline levels increase with little or no changes in serum calcium or phosphate levels. Bisphosphonates are used in the treatment of PDB but calcitonin may also help.

Radiolucencies and Radio-opacities. A. Bone Diseases

14

Radiolucencies (Tables 1–3)

Radiographic features to be assessed include the lesional size, site, shape, margins, radio-density and effects on adjacent structures (displacement of the inferior alveolar nerve or tooth displacement or resorption).

Well-defined corticated radiolucencies are often odontogenic cysts and benign tumours as they are generally slow growing and allow the bone surrounding them to remodel. If they become infected cortication may be lost and they may appear to be less well defined.

Well-defined non-corticated lesions (punched out lesions) may be odontogenic cysts, granulomas that have become infected, or more sinister rapidly-growing lesions such as multiple myeloma, malignancy or histiocytosis.

Poorly defined radiolucencies are often infections or malignant tumours.

Jaw radiolucencies may include:
■ *Odontogenic diseases*, inflammation, cysts and tumours.
■ *Non-odontogenic cysts*, eg nasopalatine duct cyst (in maxillary midline, with a characteristic heart shape), and

Procedure	Advantages	Disadvantages	Remarks
Aspiration	Simple using 18 gauge needle	May introduce infection	May confirm haemangioma. Cyst fluid protein content may be diagnostic (Protein levels <4g% in keratocysts)
Bone biopsy	Definitive	Invasive	Most commonly used
Bone scan	Surveys all skeleton	Those of any isotope procedure	Reveals areas of increased bony turnover, eg metastases; lacks specificity
Endoscopy (fibre-optic)	Simple; good	Skill needed visualization	Examines nasal passages, sinuses, pharynx and larynx but not widely available
Imaging	Reveals data not obvious on clinical examination	Specialized techniques may be difficult or expensive. Cone beam CT (CBCT) is becoming more widely used and available	See Table 2

Table 1. Investigations used in diseases of jaws. (Reproduced from Scully C. *Oral and Maxillofacial Medicine.* Elsevier, 2008.)

traumatic bone cyst (solitary, simple, haemorrhagic bone cyst) – the aetiology of which is unknown but has been attributed to arise from trauma causing intramedullary haemorrhage that subsequently leaves a radiolucency with characteristic scalloped superior margin (it rarely damages teeth).

Giant cell lesions such as the *Central Giant Cell granuloma* – initially a small, unilocular radiolucency – eventually become multilocular, and may then mimic brown tumours of hyperparathyroidism (histologically similar). Biochemistry distinguishes these entities. Other giant cell lesions include brown tumour of hyperparathyroidism, cherubism and aneurysmal bone cysts.

Vascular or neurogenic lesions include:
■ *Arteriovenous malformation* – abnormal communication between arteries and veins, or central

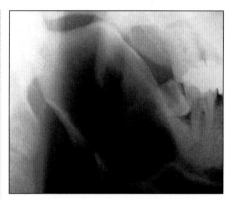

Figure 1. Oblique lateral radiograph of the right mandible, showing a well-defined corticated radiolucency. The corticated margins are continuous with the ID canal, suggesting a differential diagnosis of a lesion arising from the contents of the ID canal, in this case a neurofibroma.

Region required	Standard views	Additional views
Facial bones	OM	Zygoma
	OM 30	Reduced exposure SMV
	Lateral	
Mandible	DPT	Lateral obliques
		PA mandible
		Mandibular occlusal
Maxilla	OM for maxillary antra	Upper occlusal or lateral
	CT sinuses or CBCT	SMV
		DPT, tomography
		Endoscopy
Nasal bones	OM 30	
	Lateral	
	Soft tissue lateral	
Skull	PA 20	SMV
	Lateral	Tangential
		Townes (1/2 axial view)
Temporomandibular joints	DPT (mouth open and closed)	Transpharyngeal – rarely used
		Arthrography – almost lateral views are obsolete
	Transcranial oblique rarely used	Reverse Townes
		Consider MRI if the position of the disc is required/CT scan/cone beam CT to show abnormalities of the condylar heads or fractures

Table 2. Radiographic views for demonstrating various orofacial sites. PA = postero-anterior; OM = occipito-mental; SMV = submen-to-vertex; DPT= Dental Panoramic Tomogram. (Reproduced from Scully C. *Oral and Maxillofacial Medicine.* Elsevier, 2008.)

Chapter 14 – Radiolucencies and Radio-opacities. A. Bone Diseases

99

Lesion	Average age	Gender presentation	Site and other comments predilection
Nasopalatine duct cyst	40–60years	M>F 4:1	1% of population. Midline palate >1 cm consider cystic
Radicular cyst	20–60 years	M>F 3:2	3x maxilla: mandible
Dentigerous cyst	<20 years	M>F 2:1	L8; U3; L5
Paradental cyst	4–62 years	M = F	93% mandible 3rd>2nd>1st molar
Keratocystic odontogenic tumour	20–40 years	M>F 1.7:1	80% mandible 50% of these angles
Lateral periodontal cyst	40–70 years	M>F 2:1	76% L3; L4&5; U2 teeth vital
Central giant cell granuloma	60% <20 years	F>M 2:1	Mandible anterior to 1st molar 2x maxilla
Aneursymal bone cyst	90% <30 years	F>M slight	Mandible>Maxilla 3:2 molar region
Central haemangioma	<20 years	F>M 2:1	Mandible>Maxill 2:1 Body freq.
Arterio-venous malformation	10–25 years	F>M	Mandible>maxilla Retromolar area
Solitary bone cyst	<20 years	M>F? M = F	95% mandible 65% molar/ premolar area
Stafne cavity	>40 years	M>F	Seen on up to 1% of DPTs. Lower 7 to angle of mandible below ID canal

Table 3. Summary of cyst and cyst-like lesions of the jaws. Not recognized as a true entity = keratocyst odontogenic tumour.

haemangioma.
■ *Neurofibroma* – may present as widening of inferior alveolar canal (Figure 1).

Metabolic disorders include:
■ Osteoporosis;
■ Osteomalacia;
■ Renal osteodystrophy;
■ Osteitis fibrosa cystica (hyperparathyroidism).
All cause a loss in bone density making radiographs appear over-exposed and there is also loss of corticomedullary differentiation (loss of lamina dura, outline of maxillary antrum, ID canal tramlines).

Neoplastic lesions include:

■ *Malignant tumours*: squamous cell carcinomas (invading mainly from mouth or antrum), osteosarcomas (a symmetrically widened periodontal membrane in a single tooth may be earliest indication), lymphomas (ill-defined lesions), and multiple myeloma ('punched-out' ovoid lesions).
■ *Metastases:* from prostate, thyroid, kidney, lung and breast tumours (but 30% originate from an occult primary lesion) typically have ill-defined borders. Posterior mandibular metastases are four times more common than maxillary.

Radio-opacities

Radio-opaque lesions may be either of soft tissue

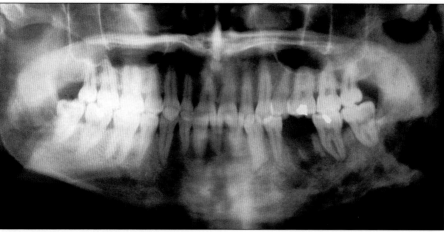

Figure 2. DPT, showing ill-defined radiolucency and radio-opacity within the left body of the mandible. Note the loss of the lower cortex and ID canal tramlines compared to the right side. This was a case of osteomyelitis.

origin or bony origin and therefore require localization with radiographs taken from two different aspects, and include:
– Unerupted teeth;
– Foreign bodies;
– Calcified lymph nodes;
– Salivary stones.

■ *Congenital and developmental anomalies*, such as torus and other bone lumps. Gardner's syndrome (colorectal polyposis, soft-tissue tumours, and skeletal abnormalities) an autosomal dominant condition caused by adenomatous polyposis coli (**APC)** gene mutation, with multiple osteomas and often impacted and supernumerary teeth and odontomas. Carriers may also have jaw radio-opacities.
■ *Odontogenic cysts and tumours* (Articles 15 and 16).
■ *Fibro-osseous lesions.*

Inflamed and infected lesions:
– *Odontogenic infections*

- *Osteomyelitis* – shows no imaging findings until the acute inflammatory reaction leads to bone lysis (osteolysis). Bone density has to fall by 30–50% to show on plain radiography and this usually takes 2–3 weeks (Figure 2). Plain radiographs, and more accurately CT (either MSCT [multislice CT] or CBCT [**Cone Beam**]) can demonstrate the osteopenia and cortical lysis (including the inferior alveolar canal and mental foramen), sequestra and periosteal new bone formation. MRI has high sensitivity in detecting cancellous marrow abnormalities. In osteomyelitis,

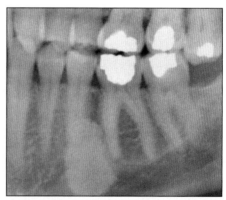

Figure 3. Section of a DPT showing well-defined increased density of alveolar bone associated with no obvious clinical or radiological pathology, diagnosed as idiopathic osteosclerosis (dense bone island).

periosteal new bone apposition causes cortical thickening and mandibular enlargement, most common on the buccal plate of the mandibular angle or body, especially in young people. Radiologically this may have a lamellar 'onion skin' appearance. Swelling of masseter and medial pterygoid muscles is common and both CT and MRI show soft-tissue inflammation, especially in the masticatory and submandibular spaces.

– *Idiopathic osteosclerosis* (dense bone island) – area of dense bone in the jaw without apparent cause or signs or symptoms, typically seen in the mandibular premolar/molar area,

Chapter 14 – Radiolucencies and Radio-opacities. A. Bone Diseases

101

which may be associated with root resorption (Figure 3).
– *Osteonecrosis*. This may follow radiation (osteoradionecrosis; ORN) or drug use (bisphosphonate-related osteochemonecrosis of the jaws; BRONJ).

Primary non-odontogenic tumours, eg prostatic carcinoma and breast metastases are occasionally radio-opaque. Sarcomas can cause osteolytic or osteoblastic lesions.

Mixed radiolucent and radio-opaque lesions

Mixed radiolucent and radio-opaque lesions are mainly fibro-osseous lesions, inflammatory processes (eg osteomyelitis, actinomycosis, osteonecrosis) and, less commonly, odontogenic tumours (mainly adenomatoid odontogenic tumour and calcifying epithelial odontogenic tumour). Florid osseous dysplasia is one of the commonest causes of multiple radio-opacities of the tooth-bearing area of the jaws.

Radiolucencies and Radio-opacities. B. Odontogenic Disease and Cysts

Odontogenic diseases may be related to the tooth or tooth germ.

Odontogenic infections

Caries, periodontitis or pericoronitis are the common oral pyogenic infections. Depending on the bacterial load and host immunity, dental pulpal infection may lead to apical periodontitis, abscess and fascial space infection, or granuloma or periapical (radicular) cyst.

Odontogenic cysts

Most jaw cysts arise from odontogenic epithelium. Odontogenic cysts (and tumours) arise from ectoderm, mesenchyme or a combination (ectomesenchyme) involved in tooth germ formation and they may be related to the site of a tooth germ, or may be associated with a tooth. There is an overall male predominance and the mandible is affected three times as commonly as the maxilla.

Clinical features

Jaw cysts are often asymptomatic presenting as an incidental finding, on radiographs, as a well-defined, corticated radiolucency owing to their benign, slow-growing nature. They may reach a large size before they give rise to:

- Swelling: initially a smooth bony hard lump with overlying normal mucosa but, as bone thins, it may crackle on palpation like an egg shell. The cyst may resorb bone and show through as a blueish fluctuant swelling. Cystic expansion is more likely to give rise to buccal rather than lingual swelling.
- Discharge.
- Pain: if infected or if the jaw fractures pathologically.

Occasionally carcinomas may arise within some cysts.

Diagnosis

Most cysts are discovered on intra-oral radiography or on dental panoramic tomography. In the mandible they, by definition, arise above the inferior alveolar canal. Unless the lesion is very large, advanced imaging is rarely required. Cross-sectional imaging allows bucco-lingual expansion to be assessed more easily, especially in the maxilla. CBCT is now the imaging of choice if required (Figures 1 and 2: Nasopalatine duct cyst; CBCT panoramic and sagittal.)

Other investigations may include pulp vitality testing, aspiration and analysis of cyst fluids, and histopathology.

Management

Enucleation (complete removal of the cyst) makes all tissue available for histological examination, the cavity usually

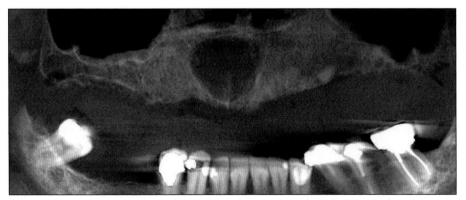

Figure 1. Cone Beam CT panoramic of nasopalatine duct cyst; note the well-defined radiolucency with intact bony margins.

heals uneventfully with minimal aftercare, but may render adjacent teeth non-vital. Marsupialization (partial removal) requires considerable aftercare and co-operation in keeping the cavity clean – the patient syringing the cyst cavity after meals. Healing may take up to 6 months and not all cyst lining is available for histopathology.

Odontogenic cysts are relatively common – most are inflammatory (55% of all) or dentigerous (22%) (Table 1). Odontogenic cysts that can be problematical, because of recurrence and/or aggressive growth, include especially the calcifying odontogenic and glandular odontogenic cysts.
■ *Periapical (radicular; or dental) cyst* is inflammatory, and the most common odontogenic cyst (75% occur in the maxilla and 56% affect upper lateral incisors). It results from pulpal infections leading to periapical infection, a granuloma, and, finally, a cyst. The epithelial lining is derived from the rests of Malassez and is thick, irregular, squamous epithelium, with granulation tissue forming the wall in denuded areas. There may be areas of chronic or acute inflammation with abscess formation. Cholesterol crystal clefts and mucous cells may be found. The cyst fluid is usually watery but may be thick and viscid with cholesterol crystal clefts. The cysts have capsules of fibrous connective tissue.

Characterized by its position at the apex of a non-vital tooth (pulp necrotic because of caries, trauma or deep restoration), there is a round or pear-shaped, well-defined radiolucent lesion with sclerotic borders, larger (often >20 mm) than a periapical granuloma, with a rounder contour, and more well-defined border. It often involves a maxillary incisor or canine.

Any cyst that remains after surgery is termed a *residual cyst* – most arise from periapical cysts.
■ *Follicular (dentigerous) cyst* is the most common developmental odontogenic cyst. It forms from the follicle of

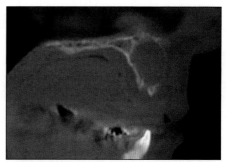

Figure 2. Cone beam CT sagittal view; note the buccal expansion and thinning of buccal cortical bone.

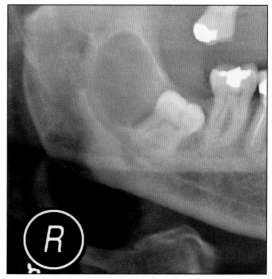

Figure 3. Section of a DPT showing a well-defined, corticated radiolucency associated with the crown of a tooth. The differential diagnosis would be a slow-growing lesion, such as an odontogenic cyst or possibly an odontogenic tumour.

Odontogenic		Non-odontogenic	Pseudocysts
Inflammatory	**Developmental**		
Apical radicular cyst/granuloma	Dentigerous cyst	Nasopalatine cyst	Haematopoietic bone marrow defect
Lateral radicular cyst	Eruption cyst		Stafne bone cyst
Residual radicular cyst	Lateral periodontal cyst		Traumatic bone cyst
Paradental			
Buccal bifurcation cyst			

Table 1. Jaw cysts. Modified from Regezi JA. *Mod Pathol* 2002; **15**(3): 331–341.

Chapter 15 – Radiolucencies and Radio-opacities. B. Odontogenic Diseases and Cysts

105

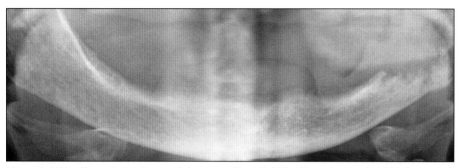

Figure 4. DPT radiograph showing a radiolucency with an ill-defined irregular margin which is not corticated. In the absence of signs of acute inflammation, a malignancy should be suspected.

Type	Decade at Presentation	Commonest Location	Usual Management
Dentigerous	3rd and 4th	Lower third molars, maxillary canines	Enucleation or marsupialization
Eruption	1st	Anterior to permanent molars	Nil unless impeding eruption
Radicular	3rd and 4th	Anterior maxilla	Enucleation
Residual	4th and 5th	Anterior maxilla	Enucleation or marsupialization

Table 2. Main odontogenic cysts.

an unerupted tooth and, therefore, the tooth crown projects into the well-demarcated cavity lined by flattened stratified epithelium (a pericoronal position may also be seen in the keratocystic odontogenic tumour (KCOT) and other benign tumours). Follicular cysts are unilocular, radiolucent, and may become extremely large (more so than the radicular cyst) but, in contrast to a malignant lesion, cortical bone is usually preserved. (Figure 3: Benign cystic lesion and Figure 4: Malignancy.)

A hyperplastic follicle, in contrast, is <2–3 mm, and neither displaces the tooth nor causes cortical expansion.
■ *Eruption cysts* are minor soft tissue forms of dentigerous cysts. They often burst spontaneously. In some cases, the teeth are prevented from eruption by fibrous tissue overlying them.
■ *Lateral periodontal cyst* is small, and lateral to a vital tooth root, often in mandibular canine and premolar regions (*botryoid odontogenic cyst* is similar except that it is polycystic).
■ *Buccal bifurcation cyst* is centred on the first or second mandibular molar, often presenting with delayed tooth eruption.
■ *Glandular odontogenic cyst* (GOC: sialo-odontogenic cyst) is rare but may superficially mimic a central muco-epidermoid carcinoma. Features include epithelial whorls, cuboidal eosinophilic cells, goblet cells, ciliated cells and mucous pools which, with expression of p53 and Ki67, may aid the diagnosis. GOC tend to be aggressive and may recur following curettage.

The main odontogenic cysts are listed in Table 2.

Radiolucencies and Radio-opacities. C. Odontogenic Tumours

Odontogenic tumours

Odontogenic tumours are rare, are often asymptomatic, and discovered incidentally on imaging (Table 1). They are generally slow-growing and may reach
a large size before becoming
symptomatic, eg:
■ Swelling, sometimes with cortical perforation. Despite some odontogenic tumours expanding rather than destroying bone, there may be local invasion of surrounding bone;
■ Pain due to secondary infection or pathological fracture.

They usually appear as well-defined corticated unilocular or multilocular radiolucencies but, unlike cysts, they are more likely to cause root resorption and buccal and lingual cortical expansion.

The majority of odontogenic tumours are benign. Management is surgical and is dependent upon the type of tumour and varies from enucleation to resection.

Benign odontogenic tumours

Benign odontogenic tumours are 100 times more common than malignant ones: most (>50%)
are odontomas, or ameloblastomas
(around 10%).

Ameloblastomas are significant since they may recur or metastasize. Composed of ameloblast-like epithelial cells arranged as a peripheral layer around a central area resembling stellate reticulum, two main histological types exist. The *follicular* type contains discrete islands (follicles) of epithelial cells: the *plexiform* type consists of anastomosing strands. Ameloblastomas predominate in the posterior mandible, presenting typically in third to fifth decades as a slow-growing, painless, uni- or multi-locular mass ('soap-bubble' appearance on imaging) (Figures 1 and 2) usually replacing a tooth and producing more buccolingual expansion and knife edge root resorption than does KCOT (but differentiation is difficult by plain radiography or CT). MRI may then help.

Squamous odontogenic tumour is rare and usually presents

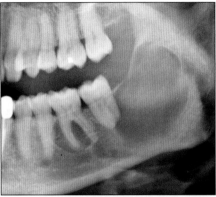

Figure 1. DPT of a well-defined multilocular radiolucency extending from the LL5 to the ramus of the mandible. Note the early apical resorption of the roots of the lower second molar. Diagnosis was an ameloblastoma.

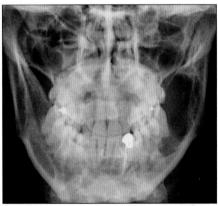

Figure 2. PA jaws of the ameloblastoma showing extensive lingual expansion consistent with a diagnosis of a solid rather than a cystic lesion.

as a painless swelling and radiolucency
between teeth which become
mobile. It may mimic periodontal disease.

Calcifying epithelial odontogenic tumour (CEOT: Pindborg tumour) – rare, benign but aggressive. Three distinct histological features are:

- Sheets of pleomorphic epithelial cells, in places, characterized by a clear cytoplasm ('clear cells');
- Amyloid;
- Concentric masses of calcified tissues.

Usually seen in mandibular premolar or molar region associated with the crown of an impacted tooth, CEOT is radiolucent with scattered calcified components.

Adenomatoid Odontogenic Tumour – is the 'two-thirds tumour' – most commonly noted in the second and third decades of life and two-thirds of cases:

- Are in females;
- Occur in the anterior maxilla;
- Are associated with an impacted tooth (usually canine).

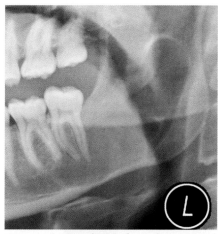

Figure 3. Sectional DPT of an odontogenic keratocyst; note the similarity in appearance to the ameloblastoma in Figure 1 but absence of apical root resorption.

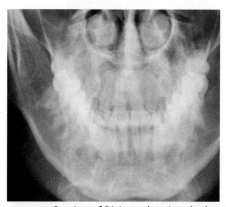

Figure 4. Section of PA jaws showing the keratocyst with little bucco-lingual expansion in relation to its size compared to the ameloblastoma in Figure 2.

BENIGN	MALIGNANT
Odontogenic epithelium with mature, fibrous stroma without odontogenic ectomesenchyme	**Odontogenic carcinomas**
Ameloblastoma, solid/multicystic type	Metastasizing (malignant) ameloblastoma
Ameloblastoma, extra-osseous/peripheral type	Ameloblastic carcinoma – primary type
Ameloblastoma, desmoplastic type	Ameloblastic carcinoma – secondary type (dedifferentiated), intraosseous
Ameloblastoma, unicystic type	Ameloblastic carcinoma – secondary type (dedifferentiated), peripheral
Squamous odontogenic tumour	Primary intra-osseous squamous cell carcinoma – solid type
Calcifying epithelial odontogenic tumour	Primary intra-osseous squamous cell carcinoma derived from keratocystic odontogenic tumour
Adenomatoid odontogenic tumour	Primary intra-osseous squamous cell carcinoma derived from odontogenic cysts
Keratocystic odontogenic tumour (KCOT)	Clear cell odontogenic carcinoma
Odontogenic epithelium with odontogenic ectomesenchyme, with or without hard tissue formation	Ghost cell odontogenic carcinoma
Ameloblastic fibroma	**Odontogenic sarcomas**
Ameloblastic fibrodentinoma	Ameloblastoma fibrosarcoma
Ameloblastic fibro-odontoma	Ameloblastic fibrodentino and fibro-odonto sarcoma
Odontoma (odontome)	
Odontoma, complex type	
Odontoma, compound type	
Odontoameloblastoma	
Calcifying cystic odontogenic tumour	
Dentinogenic ghost cell tumour	
Mesenchyme and/or odontogenic ectome-senchyme with or without odontogenic epithelium	
Odontogenic fibroma	
Odontogenic myxoma/myxofibroma	
Cementoblastoma	

Table 1. WHO classification of odontogenic tumours.

Chapter 16 – Radiolucencies and Radio-opacities. C. Odontogenic Tumours

109

Tumour type and % of odontogenic tumours	Age in years	Site	Association with unerupted teeth	Resorption of teeth	Other features
Ameloblastoma 11%	80%<40	90% mandible molar region	38% (predominantly third molar region)	39% knife edge	Multilocular; angle of mandible preserved.
Ameloblastic fibroma 2%	<20 40%<10	73% mandible molar/premolar	100%	Rare	Multilocular: less likely to destroy areas of expanded cortex than ameloblastoma.
Ameloblastic fibro-odontoma 2%	<20	Mandible = maxilla 25% anterior jaw	100%	Rare	Multilocular; very small lesions cause large amount of tooth displacement.
Adenomatoid odontogenic tumour 3%	5–50 Average 16 70% teenage	75% maxilla 90% in canine incisor region	74%	Rare	Snowflake opacities evenly arranged throughout lesion.
Calcifying epithelial odontogenic tumour 1%	30–50 peak 40	Mandible 2x maxilla Molar 3x premolar	52% rarely impacted Calcification begins	May occur knife edge	Maybe multilocular: lesion tends to extend into body rather than ramus. Less well defined than ameloblastoma.
Calcifying cystic odontogenic Tumour 2%	10–19	Mandible = maxilla 75% ant to 6	20–25%	Occasionally	Hydraulic bone expansion, expanded bone may appear perforated.
Keratocystic odontogenic tumour Commonest odontogenic tumour 3–10% of cyst like lesions	20–50	Mandible 3x maxilla			10% multiple. CT scan if sinus involved. Radiolucency in ramus not contacting any teeth most likely keratocyst. Minimal tooth displacement. Perforation of cortex may occur.
Odontogenic fibro/myxoma 3–5%	Mean 25–35	Mandible 3x maxilla Molar>premolar	5% often congenitally absent tooth rare ramus	Occasionally	May be multilocular; May destroy angle of mandible Septa intersect at 90°; may cross midline.
Cement-ossifying fibroma 40% of FCOL	15–50	80% mandible premolar and molar Maxilla, zygoma and canine		May occur	Expansion of bone equally in all directions Cortex remains intact Bowing of inferior border parallels tumour mass.
Benign cementoblastoma 9% of FCOL	<25	85% mandible 60% 1st molar 20–25% premolars		50% resorption of fusion	Only cemental lesion to be attached to root of involved tooth.
Odontomes 67%	<20	Compound: Anterior maxilla 62%. Complex: Mandible 1st 2nd molar 70%	48%	Rare	Compound 2x as common as complex.

Table 2. Summary of odontogenic tumours. Hamartomas, FCOL = Fibrous cemento-osseous lesions. Note multilocular lesions may also give rise to unilocular radiolucencies.

Normal follicle space 2.5 mm intra-oral 3 mm DPT	>2.5 80% cystic The canine has larger follicle space
Radicular cyst or granuloma	Diameter >1.6 cm or Area 200 mm
Dentigerous cysts	Lingual expansion rare
Keratocystic odontogenic tumour	10% multiple CT scan if sinus involved. Radioluency in ramus not contacting any teeth most likely keratocyst. Minimal tooth displacement. Perforation of cortex may occur.
Nasopalatine cyst Normal size of nasopalatine duct 6 x 7 mm	4:1 M:F Diameter >1cm ?cystic Normal well-defined lateral walls only
Central Giant Cell Granuloma	F:M 2:1 60% < 20 years of age. Associated with Paget's disease. Rare in ramus; usually anterior to first molar; uneven buccolingual expansion.
Aneurysmal bone cyst	90% < 30 years. Cortex remains intact even when large. Marked buccolingual expansion compared to AP.
Central haemangioma	Premature exfoliation of 1° and delayed eruption of 2° teeth. Phleboliths. Vertical expansion important feature
Arteriovenous malformation	Cortical thinning without perforation Sunray appearance: Phleboliths
Solitary bone cysts	50% > 3 cm. Few extend into ramus 70% have scalloped upper margin
Ameloblastoma *The Great Mimicker*	80% < 40 years. 10–15% unilocular 38% associated with unerupted teeth MRI better for recurrence high signal on T2 weighted images Angle usually preserved Locules larger centrally
Ameloblastic fibroma	Even when small causes buccolingual expansion
Ameloblastic odontofibroma	Small lesion large tooth displacement
Adenomatoid odontogenic tumour	74% unerupted tooth. 68% canines, 70% < 20 years, F:M 2:1
Calcifying epithelial odontogenic tumour	Frequently scalloped margin. Variable definition. Expands into body rather than ramus.
Calcifying cystic odontogenic tumour	Hydrostatic expansion. Cortical perforation 96% unilocular
Odontogenic myxoma	Soap bubble appearance; expansion and perforation May destroy angle
Benign cementoblastoma	Attaches to tooth root Occlusal film sunray appearance
Cement-ossifying fibroma	Expansion inferior cortex of the mandible

Table 3. Useful points in diagnosis of radiolucent lesions of the jaws.

Chapter 16 – Radiolucencies and Radio-opacities. C. Odontogenic Tumours

111

Sheets and strands of epithelial cells are arranged as convoluted bands and tubular structures, in which ameloblast-like cells are arranged radially around a homogeneous eosinophilic material. It presents as a well-demarcated unilocular radiolucent lesion, often with punctate calcifications. It rarely recurs after excision.

Keratocystic odontogenic tumour (KCOT) has a propensity for destruction and recurrence locally. Radiologically, KCOT usually presents as a well-defined corticated unilocular or multilocular radiolucency which enlarges through cancellous bone, giving rise to late cortical expansion, and for its size the amount of bucco-lingual expansion is small compared to other odontogenic tumours (Figures 3 and 4). The lining has a regular keratinized stratified squamous epithelium, five to eight cell layers thick and without rete pegs. Desquamated keratin is often present within the lumen and the fibrous wall is usually thin. KCOT are often multilocular, well-defined, radiolucent, usually without an associated tooth. The keratin-rich debris shows a characteristic central signal drop on MRI T2-weighted images.

KCOT is associated with chromosome 9 patch gene mutations. Multiple KCOTs in young patients should suggest the basal cell naevus (Gorlin-Goltz) syndrome – an autosomal dominant disorder also with midface hypoplasia, frontal bossing and prognathism, falx cerebri calcification and skeletal anomalies.

Ameloblastic fibroma consists of islands, elongated strands, or terminal buds of ameloblast-like cells and central stellate reticulum cells, surrounded by a cellular hyaline material. It is usually well-defined, pericoronal multiloculated radiolucent and associated with an impacted tooth, often in the posterior mandible.

Odontogenic myxoma is clinically and radiographically indistinguishable from ameloblastoma.

Odontoma (odontome) – a 'hamartoma' consisting of dentine and enamel, is often associated with an impacted tooth, classified as follows:
- Compound type (Compound composite odontomes) – multiple small simple denticles embedded in fibrous connective tissue within a capsule. Multiple lesions may be seen in Gardner syndrome;
- Complex type (Complex composite odontomes) – an irregular mass of all dental tissues.

Odontomes typically present during the second decade, are more common in females than males, and often in the mandibular premolar–molar region. Typically, they can behave like teeth: they can grow and tend to erupt, or may displace adjacent teeth. Failure of a tooth to erupt is usually the justifying reason for radiographic exposure which identifies the odontome.

Cementoblastoma is a neoplasm of cementum typically seen in patients under 25 years. Usually fused to a root (typically mandibular premolar or first molar), it is a well-defined radio-opacity with a radiolucent margin. It may cause pain which responds to NSAIDs. Hypercementosis, in contrast, is smoother, less nodular, and has a thin radiolucent margin continuous with the periodontal ligament space.

Malignant odontogenic tumours

These are generally considered as the malignant counterparts of the benign categories (Table 2).

Some useful points with regard to odontogenic tumours are given in Table 3.

Radiolucencies and Radio-opacities. D. Antral Disease

17

Antral disease

Paranasal sinuses are air-filled cavities in the dense portions of the bones of the skull lined with a ciliated mucosa, the mucus from which drains via openings (ostia) into the nose. The main sinuses are frontal, ethmoid, sphenoid and maxillary. Their main disorders are inflammatory and neoplastic. This section focuses on the maxillary sinus (antrum).

The floor of the maxillary antrum will be visualized in maxillary intra-oral films and in DPTs – where the medial and posterior wall can also be assessed (Figure 1).

Sinusitis

- Definition: inflammation of the sinus mucosa. Sinusitis most commonly affects the ethmoid sinuses, which then causes a secondary maxillary sinusitis. As a result of later development of the sinuses, sphenoid sinusitis is unusual in children under age 5 years and frontal sinusitis is unusual before age 10. Maxillary sinusitis
is subdivided into acute and chronic
sinusitis, the differential being a 3-month time period.
- Prevalence (approximate): common; (15–20% of the population at some point);
- Age mainly affected: any;
- Gender mainly affected: M = F.
- Aetiopathogenesis: cilia damage (eg tobacco smoke exposure), or impaired mucociliary clearance as when ostia are obstructed (eg allergic or infective rhinitis, foreign bodies, polyps). A
change in sinus air pressure may cause pain (eg from ostia obstruction, increased mucus production, or air pressure changes such as flying or diving)(Table 1).

- Allergic (vasomotor) rhinitis and nasal polyps;
- Viral upper respiratory tract infection (URTI);
- Diving or flying;
- Nasal foreign bodies;
- Periapical infection of maxillary posterior teeth;
- Oro-antral fistula;
- Prolonged endotracheal intubation.

Table 1. Factors predisposing to paranasal sinusitis.

Bacteria are most commonly the cause, and incriminated are:
- In acute sinusitis: *Streptococcus pneumoniae*, *Haemophilus influenzae* and *Moraxella catarrhalis*. *Staphylococcus aureus* and *Streptococcus pyogenes* may also be involved.
- In chronic sinusitis, also anaerobes, especially Porphyromonas (Bacteroides);
- In some circumstances, Gram-positive cocci and bacilli as well as
Gram-negative bacilli may also be found – especially after prolonged endotracheal intubation, and in HIV/AIDS. In many immunocompromised persons, fungi (mucor, aspergillus or others) may be involved and, in cystic fibrosis, *Pseudomonas aeruginosa*, *Acinetobacter baumannii* and Enterobacteriaceae are often implicated.

Diagnostic features

History

Symptoms can include nasal drainage (rhinorrhea or post nasal drip), nasal blockage, the sensation of swelling in nose

Location	Location of pain	Other features
Maxillary	Cheek and/or upper teeth	Tenderness over antra
Frontal	Over frontal sinuses	Tenderness of sides of nose
Ethmoidal	Between eyes	Anosmia, eyelid swelling
Sphenoidal	Ear, neck, and at top or centre of head	

Table 2. Features of paranasal sinusitis

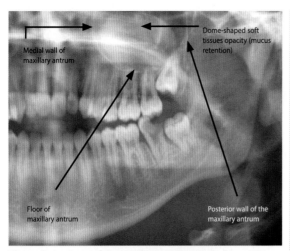

Medial wall of
maxillary antrum

Dome-shaped soft
tissues opacity (mucus
retention)

Floor of
maxillary antrum

Posterior wall of the
maxillary antrum

Figure 1. Anatomy of the maxillary antrum imaged in a DPT.

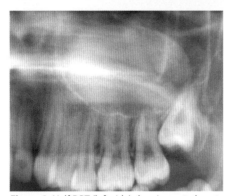

Figure 2. Half DPT (left side) showing antral anatomy and dome-shaped soft tissue opacity of a mucous retention cyst.

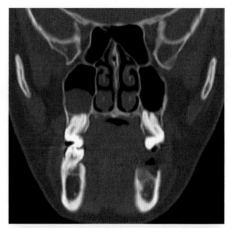

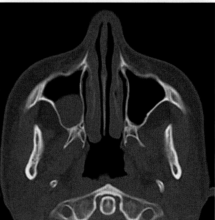

Figure 3. (a) Coronal CT of maxilla showing right- sided benign mucous retention cyst. **(b)** Axial CT of **(a)**.

or sinuses, ear symptoms, pain in teeth worse on biting or leaning over, halitosis, headache, fever, cough, malaise, etc (Table 2). Symptoms are typically less severe in chronic sinusitis.

Clinical features

There may be nasal turbinate swelling, erythema and injection (dilated blood vessels), mucus, sinus tenderness, allergic 'shiners' (dark circles around eyes), pharyngeal erythema, otitis, etc.

Diagnosis is from the history, plus sinus tenderness and dullness on transillumination. Nasendoscopy can visualize the mucosal surface inside the maxillary or sphenoid sinus in over 50% of patients. Nasal cytology with a rhinoprobe may help and ear examination is important.

Acute sinusitis is diagnosed and treated clinically and does not require imaging. If symptoms persist after 10 days of

treatment, CT is recommended when the results may affect management. Plain films are not recommended as the findings are usually non-specific. Differentiating between sinusitis and URTI is difficult. Antral radio-opacities in children under age 6 years can be difficult to evaluate since they are seen in up to 50%. In adults, a sinus radio-opacity may be due to mucosal thickening or a mucous retention cyst (Figures 2 and 3) but a fluid level is highly suggestive of acute sinusitis. Corticated opacities occurring in the maxillary antrum indicate that the aetiology of the opacity is extrinsic to the antrum, eg an apical radicular cyst (Figure 4). MRI may be recommended if there are complications such as peri-orbital infection, or to rule out malignancy.

It may sometimes be necessary to perform a needle aspiration sinus to confirm the diagnosis, and sample infected material to culture to determine what micro-organism is responsible.

Chapter 17 – Radiolucencies and Radio-opacities. D. Antral Disease

115

In patients with recurrent or recalcitrant sinusitis, cystic fibrosis and immunodeficiencies may need to be excluded.

Management

Acute sinusitis resolves spontaneously in about 50%, but analgesics are often indicated and other therapies may be required, especially if symptoms persist or there is a purulent discharge.

Intranasal steroids are helpful in many patients, although studies evaluating the efficacy have not been conclusive. Antihistamines are used for patients with significant allergic symptoms. Oral decongestants help, but typically may be used for 3–7 days only as longer use may cause rebound and rhinitis medicamentosa. Guaifenesin helps thin and increase clearance of secretion. Buffered saline lavage may help in clearing secretions. Hot steam is often helpful.

Antibiotic treatment for at least two weeks in acute sinusitis and at least three weeks in chronic sinusitis is commonly required. Treatment for acute sinusitis is amoxicillin, ampicillin or co-amoxiclav (erythromycin if penicillin-allergic), or a tetracycline such as doxycycline or clindamycin. Chronic sinusitis responds better to drainage by functional endoscopic sinus surgery (FESS), plus antimicrobials (metronidazole with amoxicillin, erythromycin, clindamycin or a cephalosporin). Open procedures including the classical Caldwell-Luc operation are generally outmoded.

Neoplasms

- Definition: usually squamous carcinoma
- Prevalence (approximate): rare;
- Age mainly affected: older people;
- Gender mainly affected: M > F.
- Aetiopathogenesis: the only identified predisposing factors are smoking and occupational exposure to wood dust.

Diagnostic features

These tumours can remain undetected until late. When they infiltrate branches of the trigeminal nerve they cause maxillary pain. As the tumour expands the effects of expansion and infiltration of adjacent tissues become apparent as intra-oral alveolar swelling, ulceration of the palate or buccal sulcus; swelling of the cheek; unilateral nasal obstruction often associated with a blood-stained discharge; obstruction of the nasolacrimal duct with epiphora; hypo- or anaesthesia of the cheek; proptosis and ophthalmoplegia consequent on invasion of the orbit and trismus from infiltration of the muscles of mastication.

Diagnosis is supported by endoscopy, radiography (Figures 5a and b), magnetic resonance imaging and biopsy.

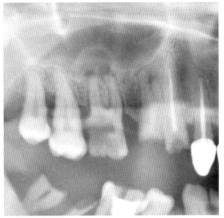

Figure 4. Section of DPT showing antral opacity with corticated margin indicating aetiology extrinsic to the antrum, in this case an apical radicular cyst associated with the upper right first molar.

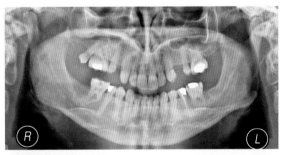

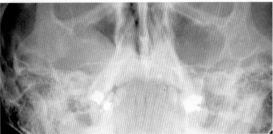

Figure 5. (a) DPT showing radiological features of a malignancy of the right antrum – opacity and bony destruction of the floor of the antrum. **(b)** Section of an occipito-mental radiograph, showing loss of lateral wall of the right maxillary antrum, a feature that is highly suspicious of malignant disease.

Management

Combinations of surgery and radio-chemotherapy are usually required.

Prognosis is poor with a < 30% 5-year survival.

Index

Note: Page references in *italics* refer to Figures; those in **bold** refer to Tables